GW00391900

Dementia: ethical issues

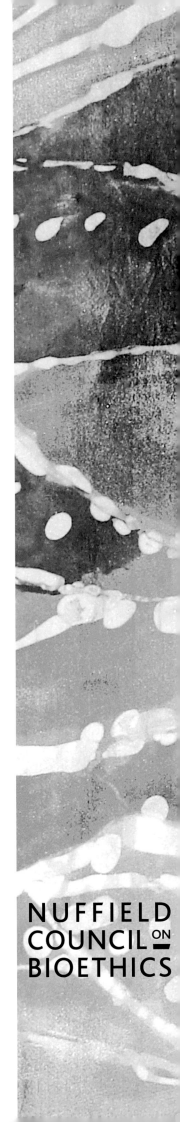

NUFFIELD
COUNCIL ON
BIOETHICS

Nuffield Council on Bioethics

The terms of reference of the Council are:

1. to identify and define ethical questions raised by recent advances in biological and medical research in order to respond to, and to anticipate, public concern;

2. to make arrangements for examining and reporting on such questions with a view to promoting public understanding and discussion; this may lead, where needed, to the formulation of new guidelines by the appropriate regulatory or other body;

3. in the light of the outcome of its work, to publish reports; and to make representations, as the Council may judge appropriate.

**The Nuffield Council on Bioethics is funded jointly by
the Medical Research Council, the Nuffield Foundation, and the Wellcome Trust**

Acknowledgments

The Council would like to thank the members of the Working Party for the considerable time, enthusiasm and expertise that they contributed to this Report. We are indebted to all those who attended and contributed to fact-finding meetings (see Appendix 1); to those who responded to our consultation and participated in our deliberative event (see Appendix 2); and to the nine peer reviewers who commented on an earlier version of this Report (see Appendix 1). We are also grateful to those who shared their work before its date of publication, including Foresight, which provided an embargoed copy of its report *Mental Capital and Wellbeing*, and Dr Daniella Wickett, who shared a draft copy of her thesis on attitudes towards advance directives

The Council would also like to thank those who provided invaluable advice on specific areas of the Report, including Dr Cesar Rodriguez and Professor Bob Woods. Finally, we would like to express particular thanks to Professor June Andrews and her colleagues at the Dementia Services Development Centre at the University of Stirling for all their help and advice.

Foreword

It is less than 20 years since ethics became a standard part of the curriculum in medical schools in the United Kingdom. It is perhaps a sign of how much attitudes within and outside the medical profession have changed that today ethical issues in health care often hit the headlines, and students in all the health professions engage frequently with such issues.

When I was working as a junior psychiatrist involved in the care of people with dementia I spent much of my time talking with patients and their families. I was not surprised by the accounts I was given of the physical and emotional stresses. What did surprise me was how frequently the problems that came up were ethical problems. Family members, for example, would struggle with questions of what is the right thing to do. These questions, far from being an insignificant addition to all the more practical difficulties with caring, were often of central importance and a cause of considerable distress. There was very little support either for people with dementia or their families in coping with these ethical problems.

The Nuffield Council on Bioethics has a distinguished track record in identifying and considering ethical issues raised by modern medicine. I had associated the work of the Council particularly with issues raised by recent advances in technology or specific discoveries from biological research. I was therefore surprised, but impressed, when the Council chose to examine the ethical issues that arise in the context of dementia. These issues are pressing not because of any specific advance in research but because of the accumulation of many developments. First and foremost among them are the increasing numbers of people affected by dementia and this is primarily due to the number of people living into old age. The biological and social sciences are leading to greater understanding of dementia, for example of the many different causes, and of the varieties of ways in which these affect people's brains and experiences. Diagnostic methods are improving. There are now drugs that can help some people with dementia. Ethical issues arise from all these developments. Any comprehensive dementia strategy must address the issue of providing support for dealing with the ethical issues that arise from day to day for people with dementia, for their carers and for the relevant professionals.

The Working Party has received unprecedented help from the public in response to its consultation on the ethical issues associated with dementia. Large numbers of families and friends caring for people with dementia wrote to us of their experiences and views. People with dementia met with us. We heard from many individuals and organisations involved in supporting those with dementia either professionally or within the voluntary sector. Researchers contacted us. We met with people developing innovative forms of support, and we discussed some of the ethical issues with a cross-section of the public at a special event arranged in Birmingham. From all this we learned that ethical issues are hugely significant. We learned too of the immense commitment, creativity, and love, all over the UK and no doubt elsewhere, that people show when dementia touches their lives. We hope that this Report, in highlighting the importance of ethical issues, will provide some impetus towards improving support for all those affected by dementia.

Finally, this Report would not have been possible without the tireless and expert help of the Secretariat of the Council who organised the events, managed the public consultation, carried out most of the drafting, and provided tremendous support to the Working Party. We thank, in particular: Katharine Wright, Kate Harvey, and Catherine Joynson.

Professor Janet Askham was a member of the Working Party until her sudden death in July 2008. Professor Askham was an outstanding social science researcher who also worked passionately on behalf of patients. She had a major interest in ageing and combined academic work with helping to develop policy to support older and disabled people. The Working Party benefited directly from her humane intelligence and her experience as well as from her research.

Tony Hope

Professor Tony Hope
Chair of the Working Party

Members of the Working Party

Professor Tony Hope (Chair)
Professor of Medical Ethics, University of Oxford, honorary consultant psychiatrist

Professor Janet Askham (deceased, July 2008)
Director of Research, Picker Institute

Mary Baker MBE
President, European Federation of Neurological Associations

Harry Cayton
Chief Executive of the Council for Healthcare Regulatory Excellence, former National Director for Patients and the Public at the Department of Health and former Chief Executive of the Alzheimer's Society

Chris Chaloner
Independent Healthcare Ethics Consultant and former Ethics Adviser, Royal College of Nursing

Dr Jim Eccles
Consultant Physician, the Leeds Teaching Hospitals NHS Trust

Professor Julian C. Hughes
Consultant in Old Age Psychiatry and honorary Professor of the Philosophy of Ageing, Northumbria Healthcare NHS Foundation Trust and Institute for Ageing and Health, Newcastle University

Dr Gemma Jones
Educator/consultant on dementia care and design issues related to dementia care; Chair, Alzheimer Café UK

Dr Rhona Knight
General Practitioner; Member of the Council

Dr John McMillan
Associate Professor, School of Medicine, Flinders University, Australia

Professor Jill Peay
Professor of Law, London School of Economics

Professor Hugh Perry
Professor of Experimental Neuropathology, University of Southampton; Member of the Council

Professor Ruud Ter Meulen
Professor of Ethics in Medicine, University of Bristol

Dr David Wilkinson
Consultant in Old Age Psychiatry, Moorgreen and Western Community Hospitals, Southampton

Terms of reference

In the light of the increasing prevalence of the various forms of dementia in the UK, and of developments in neuroscience which provide a better understanding of these conditions and of the care and treatment that can be provided, the Working Party will:

1. Identify and consider the ethical, legal, economic and social issues, including issues of social responsibility, that arise in the care and treatment of those with dementia arising from degeneration of the brain.

2. Examine ethical issues affecting individuals with dementia, carers, families, health care providers, social services and society, in particular those surrounding:

    a. decision making and capacity to consent;

    b. respect for the autonomy of both the individual and their family/carers;

    c. 'best interests' and 'quality of life' of both the individual and their family/carers;

    d. the implications of the changes that affect the behaviour of people with dementia.

3. Consider the legal, policy and educational implications of these ethical issues for the care and support of individuals with dementia and their families taking account of different cultural and social contexts, including:

    a. the implications of an 'advance directive' or 'living will' in relation to palliative care and end of life issues, produced before, or after diagnosis;

    b. the adequacy of care and support for individuals with dementia and their families.

Table of contents

Executive summary and recommendations

What is dementia? (Chapter 1)

1. The term 'dementia' describes a collection of signs and symptoms such as memory and communication problems, changes in mood and behaviour, and the gradual loss of control of physical functions which, taken together, are an indication of damage to the brain as a result of the progressive degeneration of nerve cells. This can be caused by a variety of different diseases, of which Alzheimer's disease is the most common. Others include vascular dementia, Lewy body dementia, dementia related to Parkinson's disease, frontotemporal dementia, alcohol-related dementias and prion diseases.

2. About 700,000 people in the UK currently have dementia, and this is likely to increase to 1.7 million by 2051. Its prevalence increases rapidly with age, affecting about one in five of us by the age of 85. In addition to its profound personal and social impact, dementia has significant financial implications for those with dementia, for their families and carers, and for our health care and social care systems. In the UK the overall annual economic cost of late-onset dementia is estimated at over £17 billion.

3. Dementia gives rise to many ethical questions affecting both the individuals directly involved – the person with dementia themselves together with their close family and friends who provide much of their support – and society as a whole. We now know much more about the damage to the brain that leads to the symptoms and behaviours of dementia, but we also have a growing awareness of the abilities and emotions which are retained long into dementia, despite serious cognitive losses. This increased understanding poses a strong challenge to past ideas of dementia as a 'death that leaves the body behind' and raises important questions as to the way in which people with dementia are currently regarded and respected. Yet this increase in knowledge has not yet delivered treatments which have more than a temporary effect. This lack of a 'quick-fix' solution challenges us to look more closely at how people can be supported to live well with dementia, how their experience of disability can be minimised, and the implications of this for both services and research.

4. Even with the best support, a person with dementia will experience profound effects in their life as a result of their disease. The decline in mental capacity and ability to function independently, together with the effect dementia may have on mood and behaviour, is highly distressing to the person with dementia themselves, and creates difficulties for carers as they seek to respond appropriately. The potential for frequent and serious conflicts of interest between the person being cared for and their carer or carers generates further ethical difficulties. The increasing number of people developing dementia means that many more people will be facing these questions in their own lives. This raises further ethical questions about how society supports people with dementia, and how it prioritises various forms of research into dementia.

An ethical framework (Chapter 2)

5. Those providing support and care for people with dementia face ethical problems on a daily basis: for example when balancing safety with freedom; deciding what is in the best interests of the person with dementia; and recognising that the needs of the person with dementia may sometimes conflict with the needs of others who also deserve consideration. While legal frameworks and guidelines are helpful in guiding practice and decision-making, they need interpreting and

applying to specific situations, and cannot provide precise answers to particular ethical problems. We propose an ethical framework, set out below, to help those who face these ethical problems, while emphasising that there is rarely a single 'right' answer in any specific situation. Our framework also provides a basis for the recommendations we make throughout this Report to those bodies whose remit affects the lives of people with dementia and their carers.

6.   We emphasise, however, that guidelines and frameworks alone are not enough to provide proper support for carers, care workers and professionals. Education and support in ethical decision-making, in the form of ongoing professional education, courses and peer support, must be available to all those providing care on a paid basis, and to all carers who wish to access such support.

7.   The framework that we propose in this Chapter has six main components, as set out in the box below.

Dementia: an ethical framework (Box 2.1)

Component 1:   **A 'case-based' approach to ethical decisions:** Ethical decisions can be approached in a three-stage process: identifying the relevant facts; interpreting and applying appropriate ethical values to those facts; and comparing the situation with other similar situations to find ethically relevant similarities or differences.

Component 2:   **A belief about the nature of dementia:** Dementia arises as a result of a brain disorder, and is harmful to the individual.

Component 3:   **A belief about quality of life with dementia:** With good care and support, people with dementia can expect to have a good quality of life throughout the course of their illness.

Component 4:   **The importance of promoting the interests both of the person with dementia and of those who care for them:** People with dementia have interests, both in their autonomy and their well-being. Promoting autonomy involves enabling and fostering relationships that are important to the person, and supporting them in maintaining their sense of self and expressing their values. Autonomy is not simply to be equated with the ability to make rational decisions. A person's well-being includes both their moment-to-moment experiences of contentment or pleasure, and more objective factors such as their level of cognitive functioning. The separate interests of carers must be recognised and promoted.

Component 5:   **The requirement to act in accordance with solidarity:** The need to recognise the citizenship of people with dementia, and to acknowledge our mutual interdependence and responsibility to support people with dementia, both within families and in society as a whole.

Component 6:   **Recognising personhood, identity and value:** The person with dementia remains the same, equally valued, person throughout the course of their illness, regardless of the extent of the changes in their cognitive and other functions.

What is an ethical approach to care? (Chapter 3)

Some general points about the care of people with dementia

8.   The concept of 'supportive care' is particularly helpful in dementia, in that it emphasises the need to support both the person with dementia and their family from the moment of diagnosis. In terms of our ethical values, such supportive care recognises the value of the person with dementia and is concerned to promote the well-being and autonomy of that person while also paying attention to the interests of carers. However, the 'label' attached to care is less important than the beliefs and attitudes underpinning that label. If care is provided on the basis that the person with dementia is valued as a person and supported to 'live well' with dementia, within the context of their own family and other relationships, then the label becomes immaterial.

9.   We also emphasise two particular points which we believe to be especially important in dementia care. First, we argue that **how things are done, so that people with dementia feel valued individuals, will often be far more important than the particular structure or format of services** (paragraph 3.5). Secondly, we highlight the enormous importance of families and friends in the care of many people with dementia. It is our view that an attitude of working with

families and other carers, supporting them in their own care of the person with dementia, is most conducive to the interests of the person with dementia and best recognises the centrality of relationships with family and friends for many people with dementia. **We suggest that the appropriate attitude of professionals and care workers towards families should be that of partners in care, reflecting the solidarity being shown within the family** (paragraph 3.12). Such a partnership would involve a relationship of trust between professionals and carers, based on mutual respect for each other's role and expertise.

An ethical approach to a care pathway for people with dementia

Timing and communication of the diagnosis

10. The prevailing view at present is that diagnosis of dementia should be made as early as possible. Early diagnosis has a number of important benefits, but not every person with dementia will find that the advantages of early diagnosis and disclosure outweigh the disadvantages. We therefore emphasise the notion of 'timely' diagnosis, and suggest that diagnosis is likely to be timely at the point when the cognitive and other changes they are experiencing begin to affect their lives and the lives of people close to them. **We conclude that people should have access to good quality assessment and support from the time they, or their families, become concerned about symptoms that relate to a possible diagnosis of dementia** (paragraph 3.18). We welcome the fact that improvements in early intervention and diagnosis are highlighted in the English dementia strategy and Scottish dementia priority paper but caution that the timeliness of a diagnosis will depend on the person and family concerned. We also emphasise that uncertainties about diagnosis should never be used as an excuse not to communicate openly with a person who is aware of changes in themselves and is actively seeking explanations. Respect for that person's well-being and autonomy demands an honest response. There is, however, no value at present in attempting to screen for the underlying disease processes in the brain before symptoms of dementia appear.

11. There is some evidence to suggest that people in some cultural groups may be more hesitant in coming forward for diagnosis than those from others. Although individual choices and differences should be respected, it is important, given the potential benefits of earlier diagnosis, to understand the reasons that prevent people from coming forward. We suspect that feelings of shame and stigma associated with dementia play an important part in these reasons and that their significance varies between cultures.

    Recommendation 1: We recommend that the UK Departments of Health should encourage more research to be carried out on the reasons why there is variation between cultures in readiness to come forward for diagnosis, and the role that misinformation and misunderstanding plays in these reasons. (Paragraph 3.19)

12. Whilst the principle of patient confidentiality is an important one in the doctor-patient relationship, a diagnosis of dementia has important implications not only for the person with dementia, but also for close family members who are likely to take on a significant caring role and need appropriate information and support to do so. **Professionals responsible for communicating a diagnosis of dementia should actively encourage the person with dementia to share this information with their family, making clear that the diagnosis is of importance to those providing informal care and support, as well as to the individual concerned** (paragraph 3.23). If the person with dementia refuses absolutely to allow information to be shared with others, this refusal must be honoured while the person has the capacity to make this decision. However, the professionals involved should make a careful assessment of the person's capacity, and also make it clear to the person with dementia that it may be necessary to share information

with others later, once capacity to make this decision has been lost, in the interests of the person's own well-being.

Recommendation 2: We recommend that the General Medical Council and relevant royal colleges, including the Royal College of Psychiatrists, the Royal College of Physicians, the Royal College of General Practitioners and the Royal College of Nursing, should consider ways of promoting an approach to the disclosure of a diagnosis of dementia that acknowledges the role of those close to the person with dementia, for example through the production of guidance on family involvement and confidentiality at the point of diagnosis. (Paragraph 3.24)

Information, communication and signposting to services

13. There is ample evidence that, in many cases, people are presented with a diagnosis of dementia and simply told to come back in a year's time. **It was argued forcefully in one of our fact-finding meetings with people in front-line dementia care that such a lack of information and support in the immediate aftermath of diagnosis is simply morally wrong. We agree** (paragraph 3.26). Access to supportive care, including appropriate information, emotional support, and a variety of forms of practical support, is essential for people to live well with dementia, making the most of all their retained abilities.

14. People also need help in accessing what is inevitably a fragmented support system, given the wide range of health and social services that people with dementia and their families may potentially use. We suggest that an important element will be the identification of a single individual to liaise with the person with dementia and their family, and with whom a trusting relationship can develop. **We welcome the proposal in the English dementia strategy to pilot possible models of 'dementia care advisers', whose role would be to help people diagnosed with dementia access appropriate services and support. We suggest that there is a strong ethical justification for such a role to be introduced throughout the UK as soon as possible** (paragraph 3.27).

Ongoing care and support

15. **We very much welcome the increasing emphasis on services which are flexible and appropriate to the individual, and which enable them to live well with dementia – an approach based on respect for the needs, preferences and personhood of the individual person with dementia** (paragraph 3.31). A commitment to making services as flexible and responsive as possible does not necessarily entail spending more money; rather, it involves listening to the needs and wishes of the person for whom the service is being provided and adjusting the support on offer in order to help them in what they value most.

16. The 'small things' of care are particularly important in ensuring that care is genuinely supportive of the individual, and enhances that person's autonomy and well-being. The humanity with which assistance for everyday living is offered, especially help with eating and intimate care, is crucial in helping the person retain their self-esteem and dignity, as are the manner and tone in which a person is addressed; the care taken to ensure that they participate as much as they can or wish in any decision about their day-to-day life; the trouble taken about appropriate and attractive food and environments; and access to meaningful activity.

End of life palliative care

17. End of life care for people with dementia is a matter of particular concern, with evidence to suggest that people with dementia are less likely to receive palliative medication, have

attention paid to their spiritual needs, or be referred to palliative care specialists than people who do not have dementia.

18. **We note, and welcome, the fact that the English dementia strategy, the Scottish dementia priority paper, and the draft action plan for Wales all identify end of life care for people with dementia as an important target for improvement, and that the various UK end of life strategies similarly recognise the particular needs of people with dementia. It is clear that a key factor will be the development of models of end of life care which are appropriate to dementia, and we welcome the English dementia strategy's commitment to the development and evaluation of such models** (paragraph 3.45). We also strongly agree with the National Council for Palliative Care that close working locally between those responsible for dementia care and those responsible for end of life care is absolutely crucial.

Dementia and society (Chapter 4)

Combating stigma and promoting inclusion

19. Our emphasis on the equal value of people with dementia and the importance of acting in solidarity with those affected by dementia underpin a clear moral imperative to tackle the stigma which is still pervasive in dementia. Such stigma leads not only to difficulties and delays in accessing services but also to exclusion from mainstream society. While we strongly endorse the commitments in the English dementia strategy, Scottish dementia priority paper and Welsh draft action plan to improve public awareness, we believe that information and awareness campaigns are only one part of the story. For dementia to be truly normalised, it needs to become an accepted, visible part of our society, in the same way that physical disability is increasingly recognised as part of the norm.

20. People with dementia need to feel comfortable going to a club or out to lunch, participating in the life of a church, or taking part in voluntary work, just as they did earlier in their lives. "Service providers" such as shops, leisure services and restaurants have a legal duty under the Disability Discrimination Act 1995 to make "reasonable adjustments" to enable people with dementia to access those services. However, they will often not realise this, and even if they do, they are unlikely to have sufficient knowledge of dementia to make appropriate adjustments.

    Recommendation 3: We recommend that the Equality and Human Rights Commission should give particular consideration to the discrimination currently experienced by people with dementia, and take appropriate action to publicise both the legal duties to which all "service-providers" are subject under the Disability Discrimination Act 1995 to ensure equal access to their services by people with dementia, and appropriate ways in which this could be achieved. In addition, the Disability Discrimination Act 1995 Code of Practice should explicitly address dementia with examples of good practice. (Paragraph 4.31)

The role of society in providing care and support

21. People with dementia experience a number of disadvantages in the current care system, especially in the way services are divided into 'social' and 'health' services. Many of their needs, for example for help with personal care, are classed as 'social', despite the fact that the direct cause of their symptoms is progressive damage to the brain. Under the current system, this means that support services may only be made available when a crisis has already been reached because of the pressure on social services departments to prioritise those in greatest need.

22. We argue in Chapter 2 that dementia is a medical disorder and that the needs arising out of the disorder should therefore be met in the same way as those arising out of other serious illnesses such as cancer. It is not acceptable to make people with cancer wait until their support needs have reached a crisis before providing that support and nor should it be regarded as acceptable for people with dementia to wait in this way. **The essential ethical point to be made is that the access of people with dementia to the services they need should not be determined by classifications of care. In allocating resources, and in determining standards of care, it should make no difference whether the intervention is classified as 'health' or 'social'** (paragraph 4.41).

Making decisions (Chapter 5)

23. It is a long-established legal principle in the United Kingdom that adults who are capable of doing so are entitled to make their own decisions about their health care and general welfare, even if others disagree with the decision or believe that it is unwise. It is important to remember that people with dementia, especially in the earlier stages, will retain the capacity to make many decisions, especially when supported in doing so.

24. The Mental Capacity Act 2005 (covering England and Wales) and the Adults with Incapacity (Scotland) Act 2000 provide statutory frameworks for making decisions in cases where individuals do not have the capacity to make specific decisions for themselves. Similar legislation has been promised for Northern Ireland. In all three jurisdictions of the UK, a person is presumed to have legal capacity to make a particular decision, unless the opposite is demonstrated. Moreover a person may have the capacity to make one decision even if they lack capacity to make another. Where decisions are made for people who lack capacity, such decisions must be in the person's 'best interests' (England and Wales) or have the potential to 'benefit' the person (Scotland).

Difficulties around borderline and variable capacity

25. In many cases, it will be very clear whether a person with dementia does or does not have the capacity to make a particular decision. However, there will be times when the person's ability to make a particular decision will be difficult to determine. The implications for the individuals concerned are potentially very significant: if they are assessed as having capacity they will be free to choose their own course of action (even if regarded by others as highly risky), whereas if they are assessed as lacking capacity their wishes may be over-ruled by others in the hope of protecting their best interests.

26. To avoid, or at least reduce, the problems inherent in borderline capacity, greater emphasis should be put on *joint* decision making with trusted family members. This might help bridge the gap between the time when a person with dementia is fully able to make their own decisions, and the time when formal proxy decision making becomes necessary on a regular basis. In our view, **most people do not make 'autonomous' decisions in isolation: rather they come to decisions supported by those close to them and in the light of those relationships. Joint decision making with trusted family or friends is one example of how our broader approach to autonomy can be realised in practice, and is potentially valuable, both in meeting the legal requirement to take all practicable steps to support a person in making their own decision and in supporting the person in 'borderline' cases where their capacity is uncertain** (paragraph 5.23).

Recommendation 4: We recommend that the Codes of Practice made under the Mental Capacity Act and the Adults with Incapacity (Scotland) Act should be amended to emphasise the importance of good communication and supportive relationships with families, so that joint decision making is encouraged wherever appropriate. (Paragraph 5.23)

Determining best interests/benefit: balancing past and present

27. In order to determine the 'best interests' of a person who lacks capacity to make a particular decision (or how to 'benefit' that person in Scotland), those making the decision are required to consider both the past and present wishes and feelings of the person. However, sometimes past and present wishes may differ significantly.

28. Our ethical framework highlights the importance of promoting both the autonomy and well-being of a person with dementia. We suggest that both past *and* present wishes are an expression of a person's autonomy, and that where these differ, neither can automatically be preferred. Well-being factors, such as the person's general level of happiness are also important but again cannot automatically take precedence over the person's interests in having their autonomy respected. We suggest that in such cases it will be a matter of weighing up the relative *strengths* of these claims. Factors which should be taken into account would include:

- How important is the issue at stake?
- How much distress or pleasure is it causing now?
- Have the underlying values or beliefs on which the earlier preferences were based genuinely changed or can they be interpreted in a new light?
- Do the apparent changes in preferences or values result from psychosocial factors (such as fear) or directly from the dementia (such as sexually disinhibited behaviour), or are they linked with a genuine pleasure in doing things differently?

Recommendation 5: We recommend that the mental capacity Codes of Practice should be amended to provide additional guidance on how past and present wishes and preferences should be taken into account where these appear to conflict. This guidance should emphasise that neither past nor present can automatically take precedence, but that the relative strength of the person's wishes, the degree of importance of the decision, and the amount of distress being caused should all be important factors to consider. (Paragraph 5.32)

Advance decisions and advance care planning

29. The Mental Capacity Act also makes specific provision for people in England and Wales to make 'advance decisions' to refuse treatment, even if that treatment may be life-saving. Such decisions are legally binding on professionals if they are valid and applicable to the treatment in question. In Scotland, there is no specific reference to advance refusals in the legislation, but they are potentially binding under case law. The ability to make binding advance refusals of particular forms of treatment generates strong feelings: some see them as a welcome opportunity to exercise autonomy into the future, while others are concerned that they may lead to decisions about health care that could be harmful to the person in their future vulnerable state. Under the Mental Capacity Act, an advance refusal can be revoked (and hence is no longer valid) by a person at any point while they retain the capacity to make the decision in question. An advance refusal may also be invalidated by behaviour which is inconsistent with the refusal; however it is currently unclear whether this safeguard applies at any time, or only while the person retains legal capacity to make the relevant decision.

30. While we are concerned that, in some cases, people may complete advance decisions because of the stigma and fear associated with dementia (and which we have sought to challenge in this Report), we also recognise that some individuals will still wish to avoid any prolongation of a life with dementia, however good the quality of care provided, or may have a strong wish not to be dependent on others. **If we are to promote people's interests in their own autonomy and well-being, and in particular in their *own* notion of what constitutes their own well-being, then it is right that the law should, as at present, permit those who feel so strongly to make those wishes effective** (paragraph 5.40).

31. However, we remain concerned that in many cases an advance refusal of treatment may not operate in the way that the person in fact envisaged. We therefore welcome guidance on advance refusals such as that produced by the NHS End of Life Care Programme and the National Council for Palliative Care, which provides a model advance refusal form and suggests a number of helpful safeguards (paragraph 5.41). We believe that such guidance may help those who wish to make advance refusals of treatment to formulate their wishes in a way which is more likely to be relevant and applicable at a later stage.

32. We are also concerned about the current lack of consensus as to whether an advance refusal made under the Mental Capacity Act could be invalidated by inconsistent behaviour after loss of capacity to make the decision in question. Such a lack of clarity adds to the concerns on the part both of those who wish to write binding refusals and of health professionals who have to act upon them (paragraph 5.42).

    Recommendation 6: We recommend that the Department of Health should act quickly to provide additional guidance in the Code of Practice on whether advance refusals may be invalidated by inconsistent behaviour *after* the person has lost legal capacity to make the decision in question. (Paragraph 5.42)

33. We also highlight the much broader concept of 'advance care planning' which is an important part of palliative and end of life care, and which aims to encourage all people who may be approaching the end of their lives to discuss and document their wishes about their future care. Wishes set out in an advance care plan may include the refusal of particular forms of treatment in particular circumstances. However, they may also include wishes about where the person would prefer to be as they are dying; the people they would most want to have around them; whom they would wish to be consulted about their care; and other aspects of their lives that they find most important and that may help make the end of their life as peaceful and supported as possible.

34. Where individuals wish to make decisions about their future care, we strongly support the notion that this is best achieved within the broader context of advance care planning (paragraph 5.48). We suggest that such planning should begin early, and should be regarded as an ongoing process and not as a one-off event, with any documented wishes regularly reviewed.

Pressure for assisted suicide and euthanasia

35. It is sometimes suggested that if people do not have confidence that they will be able to exert some control over their future health care at the end of life, they may prefer to consider suicide or some form of assisted dying as a way of taking more direct, personal control at an earlier stage in the illness. While one of the components of our ethical framework is the belief that life with dementia can overall be positive, we recognise that some people, when contemplating their own possible future with dementia, consider such a future, at least at some stage, as worse than death. However the present situation in the UK is that both assisted suicide and active euthanasia are illegal even where a person wishing to end their life has full capacity. We believe that in such circumstances it would be quite inappropriate even to start to consider any form of legal assisted dying in connection with dementia.

Proxy decision making: welfare attorneys

36. It is now possible in both England/Wales and Scotland for a person with capacity to nominate a 'welfare attorney' who will be empowered to take health or welfare decisions on their behalf if, in the future, they lose capacity to make those decisions themselves. A welfare power of

attorney is a more flexible arrangement than an advance refusal of treatment, in that the welfare attorney will be able to weigh up all the relevant evidence at the time a decision is needed. While the creation of the power of 'welfare attorney' has been widely welcomed, there have been well-reported concerns about the complexity of the forms, the bureaucracy involved in 'registering' the power with the Office of the Public Guardian, and the fees charged for this registration.

37. **Welfare powers of attorney are a very good way of promoting a person's autonomy interests. Indeed, they have many advantages over an advance decision as they permit decisions to be made in the light of up-to-date knowledge both of the person's clinical needs and the care options available. We therefore welcome all attempts by the Offices of the Public Guardian to make welfare powers of attorney as accessible as possible to anyone who wishes to make one, in terms of ease of completion, level of bureaucracy and cost** (paragraph 5.55).

38. We believe that, in supporting and facilitating decision making on behalf of people who are inherently vulnerable as a result of their declining capacity, welfare powers of attorney represent a 'social good' and that, as such, they should, in principle, be available free of charge for everyone. At the very least, a funding mechanism should be found in order to ensure that when a person is first diagnosed with dementia they are actively supported in nominating a welfare attorney if they so wish (paragraph 5.56).

     Recommendation 7: We recommend that the Offices of the Public Guardian in England/Wales and in Scotland actively monitor whether the current arrangements are in practice hindering anyone who might wish to benefit from appointing a welfare attorney from doing so, whether because of the cost or because of the complexity of the process. We further recommend that they work with the relevant Departments of Health to explore ways of actively supporting people to appoint a welfare attorney at the point when they receive a diagnosis of dementia. (Paragraph 5.56)

Relationships between nominated proxies and professionals

39. Although welfare attorneys have the legal authority to make decisions on behalf of the person who lacks capacity, they do not have complete freedom of action: they are obliged by law to act in the individual's best interests (England and Wales) or in a way which will benefit the person (Scotland). This may lead to potential conflict between welfare attorneys and professionals if views differ as to what course of action will be best for the person. The strict legal position is that, in such cases, professionals may only override the attorney's opinion in an emergency, with the authority of the Court of Protection (England and Wales) or, in Scotland, with the authority of a second opinion doctor nominated by the Mental Welfare Commission or of the Court of Session. However, there is little guidance for professionals as to what level of concern should trigger an approach to the Courts or the Mental Welfare Commission.

     Recommendation 8: We recommend that the Codes of Practice both for England/Wales and for Scotland should explicitly address the question of when it is appropriate for professionals to seek to override the decision of a nominated welfare attorney by approaching the Court of Protection, the Mental Welfare Commission or the Court of Session. Both professionals and welfare attorneys would then be clear as to their respective positions. Our view is that significant weight should be placed on the fact that the person on whose behalf the decision is being taken has actively chosen, in the past, to trust the welfare attorney to act on their behalf. This would suggest that others should seek to intervene only if they have grave concerns about the welfare of the incapacitated person, and not simply because they themselves take a different view of best interests. (Paragraph 5.63)

How well are the Acts working?

40. In general, the evidence we received about the provisions of the Mental Capacity Act 2005 and the Adults with Incapacity (Scotland) Act 2000 was very positive. However, even though the mental capacity Acts have the 'best interests' or 'benefit' of the person at their heart, we are concerned that, in practice, there is still a risk of a 'tick-box' culture, which may lead to the routine acceptance of unimaginative and unsympathetic decisions about a person's care. We emphasise in our ethical framework that **the difficult problems which often arise in dementia do not lend themselves to formulaic answers, and that indeed there will often be no straightforward 'right' or 'best' answer. The approach to 'best interests' and 'benefit' set out in the mental capacity legislation and Codes of Practice is very helpful, in that it encourages a flexible approach to decision making that looks at the individuals and circumstances involved in each particular case. We reiterate here the fundamental importance of approaching such decisions not only with flexibility, but with compassion, founded on respect for the value of the person with dementia** (paragraph 5.66).

Dilemmas in care (Chapter 6)

Overview of our approach

41. As we emphasise in the introduction to our ethical framework, ethical dilemmas arise on a daily basis for all those providing care for people with dementia. Such dilemmas may arise in mundane situations, but they are problematic and stressful, and those providing care often feel isolated and unsupported in responding to them. Yet the way in which they are handled may have a significant effect on the quality of life of both the person with dementia and others surrounding them. Moreover, the problems arising in dementia are complex: there is rarely one over-arching value or consideration that can be used to solve them, and hence judgment has to be applied in the light of every particular case. In view of this, our general conclusions are as follows:

    1. **Specific guidelines, rules and laws have a particular but limited role to play: they may help to set a framework pointing to ways in which problems may be resolved but they can rarely provide a definitive answer to a specific dilemma. Any such guidelines will need to be interpreted in a flexible and compassionate way when applied to a specific situation, with a focus both on the interests of the individual with dementia and on the interests of others directly concerned.**

    2. **Professionals are in a position to support both carers and care workers, in addition to facing ethical problems themselves. They should have access to ongoing education to help them in both these roles. Education in ethical decision making, however, should not be limited to those with 'professional' roles: care workers are required to respond to ethical problems as part of their daily work, and should have access to the ongoing education needed to equip them to respond appropriately.**

    3. **All those involved in direct care – carers, care workers, health and social care professionals, and volunteers – should have access to forums for sharing and receiving support in making ethical decisions. Carers and volunteers who wish to access more formal courses in ethical decision making should be able to do so** (paragraph 6.3).

        Recommendation 9: We recommend that the UK Departments of Health consider, as part of their dementia strategies and workforce planning, how all those involved in direct care of people with dementia can access appropriate education and support in ethical decision making. (Paragraph 6.3)

The use of assistive technologies

42. Technologies such as 'smart' home adaptations, telecare, memory aids and monitoring or tracking devices may play an important role in enhancing the lives of people with dementia and their close family and friends. They may promote a person's autonomy and well-being by enabling them to live more freely and more independently for longer. Concerns, however, have been raised about possible detrimental effects, such as intrusion on privacy, stigma (particularly with reference to tracking devices) and the risk of reduced human contact. All these issues have the potential to affect both a person's autonomy, for example through feeling controlled or devalued, and their well-being, for example through impoverished human relationships.

43. Where the person with dementia has the capacity to choose for themselves whether to accept or refuse a particular technology, their decision should be respected. **Where a person with dementia lacks the capacity to decide for themselves whether to make use of a particular technology, the relative strength of a number of factors should be considered on a case-by-case basis, including:**

    - **the person's own views and concerns, past and present, for example about privacy;**
    - **the actual benefit which is likely to be achieved through using the device;**
    - **the extent to which a carer's interests may be affected, for example where they would otherwise have to search for the person with dementia in the streets at night; and**
    - **the dangers of loss of human contact** (paragraph 6.12).

Balancing freedom and risk

44. Taking risks is an inherent part of our everyday lives, and a life without any form of risk is unimaginable. Those caring for people with dementia however, may often feel the need to do all they can to reduce risk to an absolute minimum. Unfortunately, minimising risk often means forgoing benefits and restricting freedom, which in turn may be highly detrimental both to the person's sense of autonomy and to their overall well-being.

45. It is clearly important that those providing care for people with dementia assess and manage risks appropriately. However 'risk assessments' can often focus only on the possible risks, without considering what opportunities and benefits are being forgone as a result. For this reason we believe that the term 'risk assessment' should be replaced by 'risk-benefit assessment'.

    Recommendation 10: We recommend that the UK Departments of Health and the four bodies regulating adult social care in the UK[1] should require care providers to consider risks not in isolation but in the context of a risk-benefit assessment. Such risk-benefit assessments should explicitly take into account the well-being and autonomy of the person with dementia, as well as their need for protection from physical harm and the needs and interests of others. The term 'risk assessment' should be replaced by 'risk-benefit assessment' in order to highlight the importance of benefits which may be lost in the attempt to reduce risk. (Paragraph 6.17)

Restraint

46. 'Restraint' includes both using (or threatening) force to make a person do something that they are resisting, and restricting their movements, whether or not they resist. Restraint techniques include physically holding a person, using straps or lap belts to keep them in a chair, locking doors to prevent them going out unaccompanied, and using medicines to calm and control

---

[1] The Care Quality Commission in England, the Care and Social Services Inspectorate Wales, the Care Commission in Scotland and the Regulation and Quality Improvement Authority in Northern Ireland.

a person's behaviour. In some circumstances, the person with dementia may understand why a particular restraint is being suggested for their own safety and may consent to its use. In other cases, however, they may not be in a position to consent, or restraint may be used in order to control behaviour that others find difficult or alarming. In such cases restraint may be experienced as highly demeaning and distressing. Yet, at times, those caring for a person with dementia may see no alternative but to use restraint.

47. For people who lack capacity to consent, the Mental Capacity Act limits the use of restraint to circumstances where it is a "proportionate" response to the likelihood of the person suffering harm. There is, however, little guidance on what constitutes a "proportionate" justification for restraint, and carers in particular may sometimes find that a lack of outside help leaves them little choice but to restrain the person for whom they care in order to get on with essential household tasks such as shopping and cooking. Regulations governing restraint in care homes make clear that restraint should be used only on an exceptional basis, as a technique of last resort, and detailed practical guidance on how to achieve this aim has been published by the Mental Welfare Commission for Scotland. Nevertheless, there is considerable evidence that restraint is much more widely used in practice.

Recommendation 11: We recommend that the Office of the Public Guardian, in association with the Department of Health, provide additional guidance to carers on when restraint might be considered to be "proportionate", either within the Mental Capacity Act Code of Practice or in the form of stand-alone guidance.

Recommendation 12: We recommend that the Commissions responsible for regulating social care within the United Kingdom ensure that detailed and practical guidance on the appropriate use of restraint in care homes, such as that produced by the Mental Welfare Commission for Scotland, is made readily available to all those working in this sector.

Recommendation 13: We further recommend that the UK Health Departments should draw specific attention to the importance of providing support to carers that will minimise the need for restraint in the domestic context, for example through guidance to health and social services organisations on needs assessment. (Paragraph 6.38)

Abuse by family and friends

48. The abuse of people with dementia by people caring for them raises particular ethical issues, because of the complex relationships and dependencies involved. While definitions of abuse differ, it is widely accepted that the concept extends beyond physical or sexual abuse to psychological and emotional harm, financial exploitation and neglect. A recent survey in the UK among carers of people with dementia found that one per cent of carers had hit or physically hurt the person for whom they cared within the previous three months. Thirty three per cent of carers, by contrast, reported behaviours such as significant levels of screaming or swearing at the person with dementia, which the authors categorised as psychological abuse.

49. The need to intervene in order to protect the person with dementia remains the same, regardless of the intent of the person causing the harm; however, the action necessary to protect the person may be quite different. While some abuse will undoubtedly be of a malicious and criminal nature, there is considerable evidence as to the role played by ignorance, stress, ill-health and exhaustion on the part of carers. Allegations or evidence of abuse must always be thoroughly investigated and action taken to protect the person with dementia. At the same time it must be recognised that abuse and neglect may be the result of unmanageable pressure on the carer. **Our focus on solidarity emphasises the need both to act to protect the person with dementia and to support their carer where the person with dementia continues to**

benefit from their care. We suggest that these concerns add further weight to the importance of providing appropriate information, advice and peer support services to all those caring for people with dementia, as highlighted in Chapters 3, 6 and 7 (paragraph 6.45).

The needs of carers (Chapter 7)

Introduction

50. A 'carer' is defined in the UK Government's Carer's Strategy as someone who "spends a significant proportion of their life providing unpaid support to family or … friends." Families and friends demonstrate practical solidarity in the care and support they provide to people with dementia, whether this is given primarily out of love, compassion, duty, a desire to reciprocate past support, or a combination of all of these. We suggest that solidarity similarly urges us (as individuals, families, communities and through the state) to support carers in their own exercise of solidarity with those for whom they care.

Joint support for the person with dementia and their carer

51. Our ethical framework emphasises the importance of giving close attention to the autonomy and well-being of carers, both for the benefit of the person with dementia and because carers matter in their own right. We also argue that autonomy should be seen in 'relational' terms: that is, that a person's sense of self and self-expression should be seen as being firmly grounded in their social and family networks. In addition, most people would wish that their carer's interests should be given considerable weight: their interests include their carer's interests. When autonomy is understood in these terms, then in order to support a person's autonomous wishes and values it will be necessary to support the whole family and social structure.

52. A diagnosis of possible dementia has implications that extend well beyond the individual receiving the diagnosis. Close family and friends, and especially the partner of the person with dementia, have to adjust to the ramifications for their own lives and come to terms with a shared future which may be very different from what they had all envisaged. **An important implication both of our emphasis on solidarity and of our 'relational' approach to autonomy is to emphasise that professional support should have a wide focus that includes helping the family to support the person with dementia, rather than being limited to an exclusive and direct focus on the person with dementia** (paragraph 7.19).

The need to be trusted

53. The issue of trust is central in any caring relationship. Most carers provide a level of care that compromises their own health and well-being, and are concerned to help and support the person with dementia as much as they are able. Given this trust-based relationship between the person with dementia and their carer(s), we suggest that **unless there is evidence to the contrary, there should be a presumption of trust in carers by health and social care professionals and care workers. Such trust is a key part of any 'caring partnership', and without such trust it is highly unlikely that the person with dementia can be given the best possible support** (paragraph 7.23).

Access to confidential information about the person with dementia

54. Concern has been expressed by many carers that professionals may be hesitant about sharing confidential information if the person with dementia lacks capacity to agree to disclosure, even where the carer feels that they need that information in order to make a proper decision on behalf of the person. The Mental Capacity Act Code of Practice sets out the legal position,

that information may be shared in such circumstances if it is in the best interests of the person who lacks capacity to do so, but suggests that carers who do not hold a power of attorney would not normally need such information as they have their own knowledge of the person to guide their decisions.

55. **The Working Party strongly supports the current legal position that when a person lacks capacity, their confidential information should only be disclosed to others where it is in the best interests of the person to do so. We believe, however, that the current guidance in the Mental Capacity Act Code of Practice on *when* it will be in a person's best interests to share information is too restrictive. Professionals should be made aware of the legitimate reasons why carers may ask for medical or other confidential information, and ordinarily start from the assumption that if a carer is involved in making a decision on behalf of the person with dementia, then they will need the same level of information as any other member of the care team. In short, carers should be provided with any information that it is necessary for them to know in order to carry out their caring role** (paragraph 7.26).

Recommendation 14: We recommend that the Office of the Public Guardian, in conjunction with the Department of Health and regulatory bodies such as the General Medical Council and Nursing and Midwifery Council, should reconsider the guidance on confidentiality currently given in the Mental Capacity Act Code of Practice, and give greater weight to the reasons why carers may need access to confidential information when involved in making decisions as to the best interests of the person with dementia for whom they care. (Paragraph 7.26)

Financial and social support

56. Caring for a person with dementia is expensive, encompassing factors such as lost earnings, paying for respite and other care, and investing in adaptations and assistive technologies for the individual for whom they are caring. Emotional and practical support is also crucial.

57. **Our emphasis on solidarity highlights society's responsibility to support people with dementia and their carers. This responsibility extends to informing carers, openly and systematically, of the social and financial support to which they are entitled: support should not only be available to those who know enough about the system and have sufficient persistence to assert their rights. We again commend the proposed role of a dementia care adviser or similar, who should be well placed to ensure that carers of people with dementia are better informed about their entitlements. We reiterate that a timely diagnosis is also important for carers, given that without such a diagnosis carers will experience significant difficulty in obtaining the help and support they themselves need** (paragraph 7.30).

Considering one's own interests

58. Carers need support in considering their own interests, as well as those for whom they care. When making a decision for a person who lacks capacity, others are legally required to act in that person's best interests. At first sight, this suggests that the interests of the person with dementia should always be placed above those surrounding them. Yet interests are often complex and intertwined. In a family, it will rarely be the case that a single person's interests always take priority: rather some consideration will be given to everyone's interests and some degree of compromise found. **Professionals such as doctors, nurses, clinical psychologists and social workers have an important role to play in supporting carers explicitly to consider their own needs and interests when weighing up difficult decisions, particularly around future care options** (paragraph 7.37).

Research (Chapter 8)

How should research be prioritised?

59. The levels of funding available for dementia research have been strongly criticised, given both the prevalence and burden of dementia. The priority given to different forms of research within dementia (such as basic research, development of treatments, prevention, social science research and research into the quality of care) is also a key issue, especially as different types of research have the capacity to benefit quite different groups. Prevention and cure, for example, both seek primarily to benefit future generations, while research focused on quality of care has the potential to benefit people with dementia in the near future.

60. We are aware of the difficulties inherent in making comparisons between the funding available for research into dementia and funding available for other conditions. Nevertheless, we are struck by the fact that the major research funding bodies within the UK do not appear to have explicit policies according to which they allocate funds between different conditions, focusing rather on research excellence and the 'importance' of the topic. While it is clearly appropriate that funding bodies support important and high quality research, criteria such as these do not, alone, ensure a just distribution between the needs of different parts of the population. **We believe that major research funders should be more explicit as to how they divide their research funds between areas of research that have the capacity to benefit very different groups of the population. Given the social and economic impact of dementia, we believe that a more explicit approach to research priorities would be likely to lead to significant increases in research funding for dementia. If such an increase were not to be matched by research applications of the necessary high standard, then active steps should be taken to develop and promote research capacity in the relevant areas** (paragraph 8.17).

   Recommendation 15: We recommend that the major research funders develop, and articulate, a reasoned basis for the division of their research funds between areas of research which have the capacity to benefit very different groups of the population. We further recommend that, if necessary, they take active steps to promote and sustain the creation of research communities capable of carrying out high-quality research. (Paragraph 8.17)

61. On the question of how funding should be prioritised *within* dementia research, we recognise that it is difficult to give one type of research priority over others. We would, however, make the following observations:

   ■ Research into the effectiveness and transferability of different models of care and support for people with dementia is relatively neglected. Yet research into these areas is crucial if people are to be supported to live well with dementia. This is particularly important given that the prospect of a real cure for dementia is highly elusive.

   ■ There are widespread concerns about the outcome measures used when assessing the effectiveness or cost-effectiveness of a particular treatment or service.

   ■ It is crucial to understand better how people with dementia and their carers live with dementia, how dementia affects them throughout the course of the disease, and how their quality of life could be improved throughout those stages. Social research in this area is an essential starting point for both the research into care models and the development of sensitive outcome measures described above. More research into the effects of stigma and how stigma can best be challenged would also be highly valuable.

   ■ All those involved in caring for people with dementia need better access to education and support in order to respond to the ethical problems they encounter on a daily basis. Further research is required on how best to achieve this aim.

   ■ Research into non-Alzheimer's dementias lags far behind that into Alzheimer's disease.

■ Research into preventative strategies appears to receive too low a priority.

Recommendation 16: We recommend that relevant research funders consider ways in which the level of funding for dementia research could be increased in the following areas: health services research into how people with dementia and their carers can best be supported to live well, how mainstream services can best be adapted to their needs, and how good practice can more readily be implemented; more meaningful outcome measures for assessing the effect of particular forms of treatment or service; research into how best to improve the provision of support for ethical decision making; all forms of research for the non-Alzheimer's dementias; and research into preventative strategies.

Recommendation 17: We particularly highlight the importance of social research in providing an evidence base to underpin better ways of supporting people with dementia and their carers. We recommend that funding bodies such as the Economic and Social Research Council, in partnership with others, take active steps to encourage further research into issues such as how people live with dementia, the nature of their experience and the quality of their lives; how stigma can best be challenged; and how those working in health and social care can best be supported in providing care which genuinely respects the personhood of everyone with dementia. (Paragraph 8.18)

Who should be involved in research?

62. Individuals with the capacity to make their own decisions as to whether or not to be involved in research may be involved only if they give consent. The ability of people with dementia to make their own decisions (if necessary with plenty of support) as to whether or not they wish to participate in research should not be under-estimated. Particular difficulties arise, however, when involving people in research studies if they lack the capacity to make their own decision about participation.

63. There are clearly good ethical reasons, based on concern for people's autonomy and well-being, for ensuring that strong safeguards are in place to protect people who lack capacity from being harmed by research. However, at the same time there is a risk that, if the procedural bar is set too high, people with dementia will be excluded altogether from research. This, in turn, would be discriminatory: it would prevent people with dementia from acting altruistically when they have autonomously expressed a wish to do so, and would reduce the chance of better treatment and care both now and in the future. **We believe that the current legal safeguards are an appropriate way of protecting people with dementia from harm. However, we believe that action should be taken to make it easier to allow those who have expressed a wish to take part in research to do so** (paragraph 8.44). In particular, we highlight the following:

   ■ The importance of good clinical trial networks which bring together clinicians and people with dementia who are interested in helping with clinical trials of promising interventions.
   ■ The importance of researchers carefully considering the possible effects of the trial on the person with dementia *beyond* the end of the trial period.
   ■ The potential benefits of people using advance decisions and advance care planning to state their views and wishes regarding their participation in research in the future. Such views and wishes could, with appropriate safeguards, provide a basis for participation in research at a time when the person lacks capacity to consent.
   ■ The difference between the systems in England/Wales and Scotland as regards the power of welfare attorneys to consent to research: in Scotland welfare attorneys have this power while in England and Wales they do not.

Recommendation 18: We recommend that the UK Departments of Health should commission research on the feasibility of developing some form of (non-binding) advance statement on research participation which could influence decisions on research participation after loss of capacity.

Recommendation 19: We recommend that serious consideration be given to enable the role of the welfare attorney in England and Wales to be explicitly extended to include decisions over research, both within the Mental Capacity Act and the Clinical Trials Regulations. In the meantime we recommend that the Mental Capacity Act Code of Practice should provide guidance on the role of the welfare attorney in decisions about participation in research governed by the Mental Capacity Act.

Recommendation 20: We further recommend that the mental capacity Codes of Practice should include clear guidance on the procedures to be followed when capacity is lost during involvement in a research project covered by the Act, to minimise the risk of research results being compromised as a result of people dropping out of research despite their initial wish to participate. (Paragraph 8.44)

64. The general principles of research governance and consent are, we believe, broadly correct. The practice, however, can place unnecessary barriers in the way of research in dementia. In particular:

■ The bureaucratic procedures around research ethics approval can be cumbersome for researchers. We encourage current attempts by the Department of Health to simplify the procedures, particularly in the context of low-risk research.

■ The ability of people with dementia to give, or withhold, valid consent to research should not be underestimated. The information provided both in written and verbal form, however, may need to be provided in a different form for people with some cognitive impairment compared with people without such impairment. Both researchers and ethics committees should adapt the informing process in a way to enable, rather than to exclude, people with dementia in making a valid decision as to whether or not to participate in research (paragraph 8.45).

Introduction

This Report is about the ethical issues that are raised by dementia.

There are many causes of dementia: the two most common are Alzheimer's disease and vascular dementia. The signs and symptoms of dementia result from the damage that these diseases do to the brain. They include difficulties with memory and other aspects of thinking, changes in behaviour and emotional responses and, as the condition develops, difficulties in self-care, mobility and speech. People with dementia often remain physically well until the very late stages and may retain many abilities.

Dementia is important because of the profound effects that it can have on the people who develop dementia and on those close to them; because it is common; and because of the high demands it places on health and social care resources. The prevalence of dementia increases rapidly with age. It affects about one in five of us by the age of 85 years and, as the population ages, so dementia becomes increasingly common. We all face a significant risk of developing dementia if we live long enough.

Dementia raises difficult ethical issues for people with dementia, for their families, friends and neighbours who provide most of their care (referred to as 'carers' in this Report), for professionals and care workers, and for society in general.

When people think about ethical issues it is often the 'big' issues that spring to mind: issues to do with the end of life, such as euthanasia, for example. But carers regularly face ethical issues in the day-to-day care of a person with dementia. Many of these issues may appear to be about trivial matters: whether forcibly to take the person to the toilet, or tell a 'white lie' to encourage the person to go to day care, or to lock the person in the house for their own safety. These, and many other day-to-day ethical issues, are not trivial for carers: it can be very wearing, and indeed distressing, to face on a frequent basis ethical problems arising from novel and difficult situations. Carers often struggle with deciding how to balance the various interests of the person with dementia: for example, their interest in maintaining their freedom when this appears to conflict with their interest in being kept safe. In addition, carers have other calls on their time and, most importantly, they need to look after themselves. How are they to juggle their various commitments? Moreover, there may be conflicts between the interests of the person with dementia and those of others outside the family, such as neighbours, or other residents in a care home.

Care workers can face a similar range of day-to-day issues, but their relationship with the person with dementia is different from that of carers and this can affect the nature of the ethical problems and the solutions. Care workers will typically be caring for a number of people with dementia and will need to balance the time they spend with each.

Professionals, such as doctors, community nurses and social workers, may need to support carers, including by giving advice on how to handle difficult ethical problems. They will also face ethical problems of their own: balancing the needs of the person with dementia and those of the carers; deciding how to communicate uncertainties of diagnosis; knowing how far to take invasive investigations; balancing safety and freedom; supporting carers whilst being alert to the possibility of abuse of the person with dementia; and deciding when to share confidential information with others.

For society in general there are the connected issues of the proper standards of care and of the resources, both public and private, that should be available. There are also ethical issues that arise in providing the appropriate legal and bureaucratic structures, for example around making decisions for those who lack the capacity to make those decisions for themselves, and in developing procedures to detect and prevent abuse. Finally, we all face the possibility that we may develop dementia and gradually lose our mental capacity to run our lives ourselves. What responsibilities do we have for planning for that possibility, in terms of making our families aware of our wishes with regard to treatment, care or research?

Our aim, in this Report, is to highlight ethical issues that arise because of dementia; to provide some analysis of those issues; and to offer some general guidance as to how to approach them. It is important, in responding to these ethical problems, to recognise that they arise in the everyday care and support of people with dementia; that no particular individual will have a single 'right answer'; and that all those involved in providing care (paid and unpaid) need much more support than is currently generally available in handling these difficulties appropriately.

We also make some recommendations as to how the ethical aspects of care might be improved. High standards of care, coupled with proper support for those caring, are crucial to any full ethical account of caregiving, and indeed high standards of care are ethically mandatory. A number of recent reports have addressed many of the wider issues around standards of care for people with dementia and the promotion of best practice,[2] and we have not attempted to duplicate their work. Rather we have focused on how our ethical framework could contribute to the promotion of high standards of care, and highlighted examples of existing services that demonstrate aspects of our framework working in practice.

It is widely accepted that if, through illness, people are not fully capable of looking after themselves, then society has duties to ensure that they receive care aimed at enabling them to have a good quality of life. This requires resources. There are many calls on the resources available both from public and from private sources, so decisions about resources must be taken within a broad context. In this Report we have therefore limited our discussion in this area to some general ethically informed principles of resource allocation and to outlining areas where more research is needed to underpin future decisions with resource implications. We also endorse the view that it is often *how* things are done, so that people with dementia feel valued individuals, that is more important than the particular structure or format of services.

Structure of the Report

The Report consists of eight Chapters and a brief conclusion. Chapter 1 provides background information on dementia for general readers (readers with more specialist knowledge may prefer to go directly to Chapter 2) and Chapter 2 sets out the ethical framework on which the ethical analyses in later Chapters are based. Chapter 3 considers what an ethical approach to care would look like, providing examples of existing practice that demonstrate our ethical framework in day-to-day care. Chapter 4 considers the issue of the relationships between those with dementia and wider society. Chapter 5 tackles the question of how decisions should be made as the person with dementia begins to lose the capacity to make their own decisions. Chapter 6 considers some of the dilemmas which occur in everyday life as a result of dementia; and Chapter 7 considers the role of carers and how their interests can be protected. Chapter 8 looks at the role of research, considering both how research into various aspects of dementia should be prioritised and how people with dementia may be ethically involved in research. Finally, the conclusion draws together the key underlying threads of the whole Report, emphasising the fundamental importance of the attitudes of all of us to dementia, and to people living with dementia.

---

[2]   See, for example, Care Commission and Mental Welfare Commission for Scotland (2009) *Remember, I'm Still Me* (Edinburgh: Mental Welfare Commission for Scotland; Dundee: Care Commission); National Audit Office (2007) *Improving Services and Support for People with Dementia* (London: The Stationery Office); Alzheimer's Society (2007) *Home from Home* (London: Alzheimer's Society); Alzheimer Scotland (2005) *This Is My Home: Quality of care for people living with dementia in care homes* (Edinburgh: Alzheimer Scotland).

Chapter 1

What is dementia?

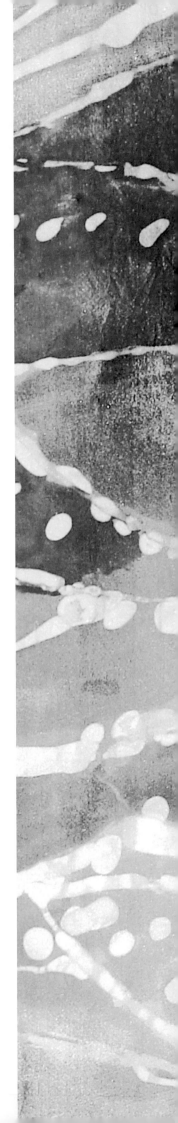

Introduction

1.1 This Chapter provides an overview of the nature and prevalence of dementia; the experience of living with dementia; the treatments and support that are available at present; the economic impact of dementia; and the scientific developments which are increasing our understanding of the physical causes of dementia. It aims to provide the necessary context for the general reader for the Chapters that follow, while not attempting to be comprehensive. We emphasise from the outset our belief that in order to tackle appropriately the ethical issues arising as a result of dementia, we need to draw both on the current state of scientific knowledge and on the direct experiences of people with dementia and of those caring for them. Neither is sufficient alone.

Nature and prevalence of dementia

1.2 Dementia has a number of scientific definitions. The term is used to describe a collection of signs and symptoms such as memory problems, communication difficulties, difficulties with organising and planning one's day-to-day life, changes in mood and behaviour, and the gradual loss of control of physical functions.[3] These symptoms, taken together, are an indication of physical damage to the brain as a result of chronic progressive degeneration of nerve cells. The damage to the brain may be caused by a variety of different diseases: while Alzheimer's disease is the commonest and best known cause, there are many others, such as vascular dementia, Lewy body dementia, Parkinson's disease, frontotemporal dementia, alcohol-related dementias and prion diseases (see Box 1.1). In this Report we use the term 'dementia' to refer to the effects of all these different causes of damage to the brain. The Report does not, however, cover temporary and reversible forms of damage to the brain. Nor does it treat dementia as a form of mental disorder, for although dementia does potentially fall under definitions of 'mental disorder' used in UK mental health legislation, it is in practice primarily treated as a physical condition which affects mental capacity.

1.3 At present, it is estimated that 700,000 people in the UK have dementia,[4] although fewer than half of these are likely to receive a formal diagnosis.[5] Worldwide prevalence is thought to be over 24 million people.[6] The likelihood of developing dementia becomes greater the older a person is: 1.3 per cent of people in the UK aged 65–69 have dementia, rising to 20 per cent of those over 85.[7] As populations in both developed and developing countries are ageing rapidly, the number of people with dementia will increase, making it one of the most important public health issues of our generation. In the UK alone, it is forecast that the number of individuals with dementia could more than double to 1.7 million by 2051,[8] while in India, China, south Asia and the western Pacific, threefold increases are expected by 2041.[9]

---

3   This is a lay definition. More detailed diagnostic criteria for various forms of dementia are set out in: American Psychiatric Association (1994) *Diagnostic and Statistical Manual of Mental Disorders* (DSM-IV) (Washington DC: American Psychiatric Association) and by the 'NINCDS-ADRDA' Work Group and 'NINDS-AIREN' International Workshop: see Scottish Intercollegiate Guidelines Network (SIGN) (2006) *Management of Patients with Dementia: A national clinical guideline* (Edinburgh: SIGN), p3, for more details.

4   Knapp M and Prince M (King's College London and London School of Economics) (2007) *Dementia UK* (London: Alzheimer's Society), pxiii.

5   National Audit Office (2007) *Improving Services and Support for People with Dementia* (London: The Stationery Office), p7.

6   Ferri CP, Prince M, Brayne C *et al*. (2005) Global prevalence of dementia: a Delphi consensus study *The Lancet* **366**: 2112–7.

7   Knapp M and Prince M (King's College London and London School of Economics) (2007) *Dementia UK* (London: Alzheimer's Society), pxii.

8   *Ibid*, pxiii.

9   Ferri CP, Prince M, Brayne C *et al*. (2005) Global prevalence of dementia: a Delphi consensus study *The Lancet* **366**: 2112–7. See also Rodriguez JJL, Ferri CP, Acosta D *et al*. (2008) Prevalence of dementia in Latin America, India and China: a population-based cross-sectional survey *The Lancet* **372**: 464–74, where it is argued that the estimates for India, in particular, may understate dementia prevalence.

1.4 It should also be noted that, despite its strong association with old age, dementia is not solely a disease of old age. Fifteen thousand people under the age of 65 living in the UK are estimated to have dementia, representing 2.2 per cent of the total number of people with dementia.[10] People with Down's syndrome face an increased risk of early-onset dementia, with an estimated prevalence of around nine per cent for those aged 40–49, and 36 per cent for those aged 50–59.[11]

Box 1.1: Types of dementia

There are approximately 100 types of dementia, the most common being Alzheimer's disease (estimated to make up 62 per cent of cases in the UK), vascular dementia (17%), dementia with Lewy bodies (4%), frontotemporal dementia (2%) and Parkinson's disease (2%).[12] Less common causes are Huntington's disease, alcohol-related dementias, prion diseases and dementia resulting from syphilis. It has been estimated that ten per cent of cases are of mixed origin, for example incorporating aspects of both Alzheimer's disease and vascular dementia.[13] These figures are not, however, universally accepted: there is significant dispute, for example, over the prevalence of Lewy body dementia,[14] and post-mortem studies of donated brains suggest that many more people may, in fact, have had 'mixed' dementias than is recognised in clinical practice.[15]

Alzheimer's disease
During the course of Alzheimer's disease, excessive and abnormally folded proteins accumulating in the brain result in the formation of protein 'plaques' around neurones and 'tangles' inside neurones, leading to the death of these brain cells, particularly in the region responsible for memory. The levels of neurotransmitters (chemical 'messengers') are also affected, disrupting communication within the brain. A combination of factors including age, genetic inheritance, environmental factors, diet and overall general health contribute to the onset and progression of the disease.

Vascular dementia
A stroke or a series of small strokes may cause damage to the network of blood vessels (the vascular system) that transport blood within the brain. The resulting disruptions in the supply of oxygen (which is transported in the blood) can lead to the death of brain cells, resulting in the symptoms of this type of dementia. Risk factors for vascular dementia include high blood pressure, heart problems, high cholesterol and diabetes.

The type of permanent brain damage caused by the interruption in the supply of blood to the brain during a stroke depends on which area of the brain has been damaged. 'Single-infarct' vascular dementia is caused by a single stroke that results in death of the brain cells in one, relatively large, area. 'Multi-infarct' vascular dementia is caused by a series of small strokes over time which cause death to brain cells in many relatively small areas, but which may not necessarily be noticed at the time by the individual experiencing them.

Vascular dementia may also be a result of 'small vessel disease' (also known as 'sub-cortical vascular dementia', or Binswanger's disease), in which blood vessels lying deep in the brain become damaged.

Dementia with Lewy bodies (DLB) and Parkinson's disease dementia (PDD)
Lewy bodies are spherical protein deposits that build up in brain cells, interfere with the chemical 'messengers' in the brain, and disrupt the brain's normal functioning. The precise mechanisms by which the Lewy bodies cause damage in the brain are not yet well understood.

Lewy bodies are also found in the brains of people with Parkinson's disease, and a significant number of people with Parkinson's disease will also go on to develop dementia.[16] The relationship between DLB and PDD is complex: it is thought that while the two conditions are part of the same continuum, they produce different signs and symptoms as a result of the different distribution of Lewy bodies in the brain.

---

[10] Knapp M and Prince M (King's College London and London School of Economics) (2007) *Dementia UK* (London: Alzheimer's Society), pxiii.

[11] Prasher VP (1995) Age specific prevalence, thyroid dysfunction and depressive symptomatology in adults with Down syndrome and dementia *International Journal of Geriatric Psychiatry* **10**: 25–31.

[12] Knapp M and Prince M (King's College London and London School of Economics) (2007) *Dementia UK* (London: Alzheimer's Society), p29.

[13] *Ibid*.

[14] McKeith IG, Galasko D, Kosaka K *et al.* (1996) Consensus guidelines for the clinical and pathologic diagnosis of dementia with Lewy bodies (DLB): report of the Consortium on DLB International Workshop Neurology **47**: 1113–24; and Serby M and Almiron N (2005) Dementia with Lewy bodies: an overview *Annals of Long-Term Care* **13(2)**: 20–2.

[15] Neuropathology Group of the Medical Research Council Cognitive Function and Ageing Study (2001) Pathological correlates of late-onset dementia in a multicentre, community-based population in England and Wales *The Lancet* **357**: 169–75.

[16] One estimate is that people with Parkinson's disease who reach the age of 90 have an 80–90 per cent risk of developing dementia: Buter TC, van den Hout FE, Matthews JP *et al.* (2008) Dementia and survival in Parkinson's disease: a 12-year population study *Neurology* **70**: 1017–22.

> **Frontotemporal dementia (FTD)**
> A rarer form of dementia is frontotemporal dementia, a term covering a range of conditions including Pick's disease, frontal lobe degeneration and dementia associated with motor neurone disease. It is caused by damage to the frontal lobe or temporal lobe areas of the brain, and there may be a family history of the disease in up to half of all cases. However, there are a number of different genetic mutations involved, all of which result in abnormalities in the production of proteins including tau, progranulin, TDP-43 and ubiquitin. Although symptoms vary between different individuals, damage characteristically appears in the front part of the brain, initially affecting mood and behaviour more than memory.
>
> **Rarer causes of dementia**
> There are many other rarer causes of dementia, including progressive supranuclear palsy, Huntington's disease, prion diseases such as Creutzfeldt-Jakob disease (CJD), and dementia associated with alcohol, HIV, multiple sclerosis and syphilis. A link has been suggested between head injury and later development of dementia, although this remains controversial.[17]
>
> **Inherited dementias**
> The most common forms of dementia are 'sporadic': that is, they occur in no particular pattern and are likely to be a result of interaction between environmental factors and the genetic make-up of the individual. A small proportion of dementias, however, have a strong genetic component. In Alzheimer's disease, these strongly inherited forms are very rare, accounting for less than one in 1,000 of Alzheimer's cases. Other rare inherited dementias include a form of frontotemporal dementia called 'frontotemporal dementia with Parkinsonism-17', familial British/Danish dementia, and a prion disease called Gerstmann-Straussler-Scheinker disease.
>
> For more detail on the different forms of dementia see the Alzheimer's Society's factsheets at www.alzheimers.org.uk/factsheets.

Current treatments for dementia

1.5 At present, the treatments available for dementia cannot reverse the underlying degeneration of brain cells, although they may temporarily improve or delay decline in cognitive function. At the time of writing, four drugs are licensed for use in the UK: three 'cholinesterase inhibitors' (donepezil, rivastigmine and galantamine) are licensed for mild to moderate Alzheimer's disease, while a fourth drug, memantine, is licensed for moderate to severe Alzheimer's disease. Rivastigmine is also licensed for dementia associated with Parkinson's disease. The National Institute for Health and Clinical Excellence (NICE) has recommended only limited use of the cholinesterase inhibitors within the NHS in England and Wales, because of concerns about their cost-effectiveness (see Box 1.2), and has not recommended the use of memantine outside clinical studies. Treatment for vascular dementia includes routine medications used in generalised vascular disease such as drugs to reduce high blood pressure and high blood cholesterol levels, while no medicines are currently licensed for the specific treatment of other dementias.[18]

1.6 Guidelines issued in 2006 by the European Federation of Neurological Societies (EFNS) cited evidence that cholinesterase inhibitors had a "modest beneficial impact on neuropsychiatric and functional outcomes" for at least one year and recommended that their use for Alzheimer's disease should be considered at the point of diagnosis, as should memantine for people with moderate to severe Alzheimer's disease.[19] Similar recommendations have been made in North America.[20] The EFNS guidelines do, however, emphasise that "realistic expectations" for their treatment effect should be discussed with the person with dementia.[21] On the non-Alzheimer's dementias, the EFNS guidelines suggest that cholinesterase inhibitors "may be considered" for people with mild to moderate vascular dementia, dementia with Lewy bodies and dementia

---

[17] Jellinger KA (2004) Head injury and dementia *Current Opinion in Neurology* **17:** 719–23.

[18] Waldemar G, Dubois B, Emre M *et al.* (2007) Recommendations for the diagnosis and management of Alzheimer's disease and other disorders associated with dementia: EFNS guideline *European Journal of Neurology* **14:** e1–e26 at e15.

[19] *Ibid*, e11–e13.

[20] See, for example, the recommendations resulting from the third Canadian Consensus Conference on the Diagnosis and Treatment of Dementia 2006, reported in Hogan DB, Bailey P, Carswell A *et al.* (2007) Management of mild to moderate Alzheimer's disease and dementia *Alzheimer's & Dementia* **3(4):** 355–84; American Academy of Neurology (2001) *AAN Guideline Summary for Clinicians: Detection, diagnosis and management of dementia* (St. Paul, Minnesota: AAN).

[21] Waldemar G, Dubois B, Emre M *et al.* (2007) Recommendations for the diagnosis and management of Alzheimer's disease and other disorders associated with dementia: EFNS guideline *European Journal of Neurology* **14:** e1–e26 at e12 and e13.

associated with Parkinson's disease, but again that expectations regarding their treatment effect should be "realistic."[22]

1.7 While the role of medicines in treating dementia is currently relatively limited, support such as information and advice, psychological therapies to improve confidence, practical help in the home, and assistive technologies have an important role to play in improving the quality of life and promoting independence for people with dementia. Detailed guidance on forms of care and support which may benefit people with dementia was published in 2006 by the Scottish Intercollegiate Guidelines Network (SIGN)[23] and by NICE and the Social Care Institute for Excellence (SCIE) for England and Wales.[24] Although the NICE 'technology appraisal' of the medicines described with respect to Alzheimer's disease above has been criticised by many, this NICE/SCIE 'clinical guideline', which makes detailed recommendations in much wider aspects of dementia care, has been widely welcomed.[25] A summary of the NICE/SCIE and SIGN guidelines on drug and non-drug treatments, incorporating also the NICE technology appraisal, is given in the boxes below (see also Box 3.1 for NICE/SCIE guidelines on social care support).

Box 1.2: NICE recommendations on treatments for dementia, associated symptoms and co-existing mental disorders

Non-drug treatments for dementia: Everyone with mild-to-moderate dementia should have the opportunity to join in a structured group cognitive stimulation programme.

Drugs for cognitive symptoms of Alzheimer's disease: Cholinesterase inhibitors should be used only for those with moderate disease, and should be started by a specialist in dementia care. A person's previous cognitive abilities (whether particularly high or low) should be taken into account when assessing their disease as 'moderate', as should fluency in the language in which the assessments are being made. The restriction of these drugs to moderate disease is made on cost-effective grounds as they are known to have some beneficial effect in early disease. Memantine should only be given to those with moderately severe to severe Alzheimer's disease as part of well-designed clinical studies.

Drugs for cognitive symptoms of non-Alzheimer's dementias: Cholinesterase inhibitors and memantine are not recommended for cognitive decline in vascular dementia, and further research has been recommended in connection with dementia with Parkinson's disease.

Interventions for non-cognitive symptoms and behaviour that challenges: These symptoms and behaviours include hallucinations, delusions, anxiety, aggressive behaviour, sexual disinhibition, apathy and shouting. Medication should be considered in the first instance only if there is severe distress or immediate risk of harm. An early assessment should be offered to identify factors that may be influencing the behaviour such as pain, side-effects of other medication, environmental factors and psychosocial factors. The person's behaviour should be analysed in conjunction with carers and care workers, and individual care plans developed. For agitation, options such as aromatherapy, animal-assisted therapy, therapeutic use of music or dancing and massage should be considered.

Anti-psychotic drugs should only be used where the symptoms are severe and where risks and benefits have been fully considered and discussed on an individual basis. Cholinesterase inhibitors may be used for such symptoms for people with dementia with Lewy bodies, or for those with Alzheimer's disease where neither non-drug approaches nor anti-psychotics have been appropriate or effective. They should not, however, be prescribed for vascular dementia.

Co-existing emotional disorders: People with dementia should be assessed and monitored for depression or anxiety, and psychosocial interventions such as cognitive behavioural therapy considered. Therapies such as reminiscence therapy, multisensory stimulation, animal-assisted therapy and exercise should be available. Anti-depressant drugs may be considered after risk-benefit analysis.

NICE/SCIE (2006) *Dementia: Supporting people with dementia and their carers in health and social care*, NICE Clinical Guideline 42 (London: NICE and SCIE), citing: NICE (2007) *Donepezil, Galantamine, Rivastigmine (Review) and Memantine for the Treatment of Alzheimer's Disease (Amended)*, NICE Technology Appraisal Guidance 111 (London: NICE); NICE (2006) *Parkinson's Disease: Diagnosis and management in primary and secondary care*, NICE Clinical Guideline 35 (London: NICE).

---

[22] *Ibid*, e14.
[23] SIGN (2006) *Management of Patients with Dementia: A national clinical guideline, SIGN Clinical Guideline* 86 (Edinburgh: SIGN).
[24] NICE/SCIE (2006) *Dementia: Supporting people with dementia and their carers in health and social care*, NICE Clinical Guideline 42 (London: NICE and SCIE).
[25] See, for example, Downs M and Bowers B (2008) Caring for people with dementia *British Medical Journal* **336**: 225–6.

> **Box 1.3: SIGN guidance on management of people with dementia**
>
> **Non-pharmacological interventions:**
>
> - Behaviour management can be used to reduce depression in people with dementia.
> - Those providing care should receive comprehensive training on interventions that are effective for people with dementia.
> - Cognitive stimulation should be offered to individuals with dementia.
> - Environmental design is important in minimising restlessness, anxiety and disorientation in people with dementia living in institutions.
> - A combination of structured exercise and conversation may help maintain mobility.
> - Recreational activities should be introduced to enhance quality of life and well-being.
>
> **Pharmacological interventions (based on clinical effectiveness but not cost-effectiveness):**
>
> - Donepezil can be used to treat both cognitive decline and the management of non-cognitive symptoms such as psychotic symptoms in people with Alzheimer's disease.
> - Galantamine can be used to treat cognitive decline in people with Alzheimer's disease and with mixed dementias, and for non-cognitive symptoms in people with Alzheimer's disease.
> - Rivastigmine can be used to treat cognitive decline and for the management of non-cognitive symptoms in people with Alzheimer's disease and dementia with Lewy bodies.
> - There is currently insufficient evidence to recommend the use of memantine.
> - If necessary, conventional anti-psychotics may be used with caution, given their side-effects, to treat non-cognitive symptoms of dementia such as delusions, hallucinations and aggression.
>
> SIGN (2006) *Management of Patients with Dementia: A national clinical guideline*, SIGN Clinical Guideline 86 (Edinburgh: SIGN).

The experience of dementia

Experiencing the symptoms of dementia

1.8 Dementia is widely seen as being synonymous with memory problems. This perception, however, is far from adequate. Some degree of memory impairment is an inevitable part of normal ageing and dementia is more than forgetfulness or poor memory. The symptoms of dementia include: more profound memory impairment which is not significantly improved either by the giving of 'cues' or through repetition; changes in attention, judgment and awareness; increasing difficulties in communication; visuo-spatial difficulties; and changes in speed of action and response. Changes in mood and behaviour, such as unpredictable anger and aggression, depression and apathy, are also strongly associated with dementia. While some of these behavioural changes, such as inappropriate and disinhibited social behaviour, have been clearly associated with the physical damage to particular parts of the brain,[26] there are currently differences of opinion as to the extent to which others may be caused, or exacerbated, by the frustrations and difficulties associated with dementia, as much as by the physical effects of the underlying disease itself.[27]

1.9 There are vivid descriptions by people with dementia of their own experience of these early stage symptoms. Malcolm Pointon, for example, a musician with early-onset dementia, wrote in his diary:

"Mind in a fog today ... thoughts and actions slipping from my grasp ... kept close to Barbara in the shops ... just didn't want to talk ... head full of cotton wool."[28]

Carers have also commented on distressing changes in behaviour:

"There was something I said to him and he went berserk, turned very nasty ... It wasn't like him."[29]

---

[26] See, for example, Shulman KI (1997) Disinhibition syndromes, secondary mania and bipolar disorder in old age *Journal of Affective Disorders* **46(3)**: 175–82.

[27] See, for example, James I and Stephenson M (2007) Behaviour that challenges us: the Newcastle support model *Journal of Dementia Care* **15(5)**: 19–22; Graham Stokes (2008) *And Still the Music Plays: Stories of people with dementia* (London: Hawker Publications).

[28] Extracts provided by Malcolm's widow, Barbara Pointon.

[29] Alzheimer's Society (2008) *Dementia: Out of the shadows* (London: Alzheimer's Society), p17.

"It was the same when he used to get into a rage, I knew it wasn't him [...] you've got to accept that it's not him. He would never have raised his voice to me at all. He was the most amiable of chaps." [30]

1.10 The different symptoms progress with time, but at a variable rate, and according to the regions of the brain affected by the underlying disease. The progression of Alzheimer's disease is often divided into three stages: early stage ('mild'), middle stage ('moderate') and late stage ('severe') Alzheimer's disease. This is a very simple division, not always related to the degree of disability the person is experiencing, and there are many further subdivisions that can be identified. While individuals' experiences of dementia will clearly vary considerably, the three stages can be used to provide a helpful summary of the kind of difficulties people are likely to experience as their Alzheimer's disease progresses. [31] During the earlier stages, the person is likely to experience memory loss, difficulty learning new things or making decisions, some degree of disorientation and bewilderment, and social withdrawal. The middle stages are associated with more serious disorientation, for example getting muddled about day and night, getting lost, and putting themselves at risk by forgetting to turn off household appliances; with increasing difficulty recognising family and friends; and also with problems with visual perception which may have a very significant effect on their ability to function independently. Finally, in the later stages, the person is likely to have difficulties with swallowing and eating, lose control over bodily functions and lose all, or virtually all, of their speech.

1.11 Other forms of dementia tend not to be characterised into formalised 'stages' in quite the same way. Some people with vascular dementia may experience a fairly gradual decline in their abilities, while others may find that they remain steady for some considerable time and then suddenly decline as the result of another stroke. Those with frontotemporal dementia tend first to experience behavioural changes associated with damage to the front part of the brain, including uncharacteristic rudeness and selfishness, along with loss of inhibition and the development of obsessive behaviour, and then later develop symptoms more similar to those of Alzheimer's disease. A person with dementia with Lewy bodies, on the other hand, is more likely in the earlier stages to experience visual hallucinations, have difficulty judging distances (leading to falls) and experience some of the physical symptoms of Parkinson's disease such as slowness of movement and tremors. Later, again, the symptoms are likely to develop on a similar basis to Alzheimer's disease. [32]

1.12 The use of the terms 'mild', 'moderate' and 'severe' Alzheimer's disease is often associated with a person's abilities in cognitive testing, particularly using the 'Mini-Mental State Examination' (MMSE), a widely used eleven-question measure that tests five areas of cognitive ability with a maximum total score of 30. [33] Scores of 20–24/26 using this test are taken to indicate mild disease, 10–19 moderate disease and less than ten severe disease. [34] However, it has been shown that many of the behaviours associated with dementia that cause particular difficulty or distress to carers,

---

[30] HealthTalkOnline (2009) Interview with a carer trying to accept that her husband's hostile behaviour towards her was a symptom of his illness, available at: www.healthtalkonline.org/Nerves_and_brain/Carers_of_people_with_dementia/Topic/2107/Interview/824/Clip/3586/.

[31] See, for example, Alzheimer Scotland (2006) *About Dementia: Some facts and figures*, Information Sheet 16, available at: www.alzscot.org/downloads/dementiafactsheet.pdf; Alzheimer's Society (2008) *The Progression of Dementia*, Factsheet 458, (London: Alzheimer's Society) available at: www.alzheimers.org.uk/factsheet/458.

[32] Alzheimer's Society (2008) *The Progression of Dementia*, Factsheet 458 (London: Alzheimer's Society), available at: www.alzheimers.org.uk/factsheet/458.

[33] Folstein MF, Folstein SE and McHugh PR (1975) "Mini-Mental State": a practical method for grading the cognitive state of patients for the clinician *Journal of Psychiatric Research* **12(3)**: 189–98.

[34] There is no agreed cut off for 'mild' dementia: Kipps and Hodges suggest 24 is widely regarded as abnormal (Kipps CM and Hodges JR (2008) Clinical cognitive assessment, in *Oxford Textbook of Old Age Psychiatry*, Jacoby R, Oppenheimer C, Dening T and Thomas A (Editors) (Oxford: Oxford University Press), pp155–63), while the Alzheimer's Society suggests that people with Alzheimer's usually score 26 or less (Alzheimer's Society (2008) *The Mini Mental State Examination (MMSE)*, Factsheet 436 (London: Alzheimer's Society), available at: http://alzheimers.org.uk/factsheet/436).

such as various forms of aggressive behaviour, anxiety, 'trailing' a carer at all times, and increased or apparently aimless walking, do not have a direct association with particular stages of cognitive decline.[35] Rather, these behaviours occur in different individuals over a very wide range of levels of cognitive impairment, highlighting the importance of considering the needs of each individual at a particular point in time without relying on broad-brush characterisations of the 'stage' of their dementia.

1.13 Research in England and Wales published in 2008 suggested that, on average, a person will live for four and a half years after developing symptoms of dementia.[36] Survival times do, however, depend significantly both on the person's state of general health and on their age at onset, with some people living with dementia for up to ten years.[37] In the 2008 study those aged 65–69 lived on average for a further 10.7 years, compared with those over 90 at onset, who lived on average another 3.8 years.[38] An American study looking at survival with different forms of dementia found that on average people with vascular dementia lived 3.9 years after the onset of their symptoms, those with Alzheimer's disease 7.1 years and those with mixed dementias 5.4 years.[39] The diagram below gives a broad indication of how Alzheimer's disease may gradually affect a person's ability to carry out day-to-day activities, although, as emphasised above, there will be significant variation between individuals, and indeed individuals may experience significant day-to-day variation in their own symptoms.

Box 1.4: How 'activities of daily living' become more difficult as dementia progresses[40]

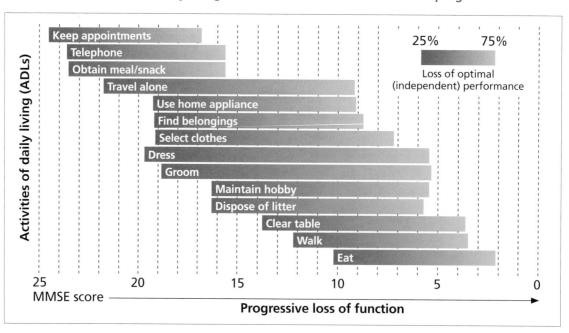

35 Hope T, Keene J, Fairburn CG, Jacoby R and McShane R (1999) Natural history of behavioural changes and psychiatric symptoms in Alzheimer's disease: a longitudinal study *British Journal of Psychiatry* **174**: 39–44.

36 Xie J, Brayne C, Matthews FE *et al.* (2008) Survival times in people with dementia: analysis from population based cohort study with 14 year follow-up *British Medical Journal* **336**: 258–62.

37 Alzheimer's Society (2008) *The Later Stages of Dementia*, Factsheet 417 (London: Alzheimer's Society), available at: www.alzheimers. org.uk/factsheet/417.

38 Xie J, Brayne C, Matthews FE *et al.* (2008) Survival times in people with dementia: analysis from population based cohort study with 14 year follow-up *British Medical Journal* **336**: 258–62. The 'average' figure cited is the median survival time of the 356 people who developed dementia and died during the 14 year period of the study (based on 13,000 people over the age of 65 at the start of the study). Participants were screened and assessed every two to four years for dementia, with onset of dementia estimated as being the midpoint between the last follow-up without dementia and the first follow-up with dementia.

39 Fitzpatrick AL, Kuller LH, Lopez OL, Kawas CH and Jagust W (2005) Survival following dementia onset: Alzheimer's disease and vascular dementia *Journal of the Neurological Sciences* **229–30**: 43–9.

40 Adapted from Galasko D, Bennett D, Sano M *et al.* (1997) An inventory to assess activities of daily living for clinical trials in Alzheimer's disease *Alzheimer Disease and Associated Disorders* **11 (Supplement 2)**: S33–9.

1.14 It is easy to characterise dementia simply as a list of things the person can no longer do. This approach, however, is strongly contested by some, such as academics at the Bradford Dementia Group, who warn against this 'deficit model' of dementia and argue that it is more fruitful to think of dementia as a 'disability', focusing on what a person *can* still do and enjoy, and adapting the environment in which the person lives to enhance these abilities and opportunities.[41] The diagram above demonstrates how a person's ability to function independently will gradually be reduced; but a rather different picture would emerge if the impact of some degree of practical help and appropriate environmental adaptations were included. Moreover, it should be noted that while 'optimal' performance of many day-to-day tasks may be affected relatively early on, some degree of ability in many areas is retained long into the progress of the dementia.[42]

1.15 Research carried out by the Alzheimer's Association in America suggests that people with early-stage dementia strongly support this 'disability' approach to dementia.[43] Those participating in a series of 'town-hall meetings' organised by the Association emphasised the importance to them of focusing on the things that they could do, and on learning to forge a new life with their retained abilities – an approach echoed by people with dementia writing in recent publications from organisations such as the Joint Dementia Initiative (JDI) in Falkirk, and Alzheimer Scotland.[44] A number of those participating in the Alzheimer's Association research also highlighted the effect the process of diagnosis had on their sense of self-esteem and self-worth: although the complex nature of dementia may make a lengthy diagnostic process inevitable, they felt that the insensitive way tests were often administered could emphasise this sense of deficit, making the individual feel that they were personally 'failing', rather than receiving a medical diagnosis:

"They put me through the whole rigmarole, a four-hour test that I came out of feeling like a total idiot. You come out thinking, 'Where am I? Who am I?'" [45]

The report's authors went on to conclude that "those with early-stage Alzheimer's seek to be defined not by the memory loss and functional decline they have experienced, but rather by their remaining abilities." [46]

1.16 While it is clearly harder to obtain the views of those with more severe dementia in the same way as those in the very early stages, accounts such as the audio-diary kept by an American academic, Cary Henderson, several years after his diagnosis of Alzheimer's disease, provide further support for the disability approach, suggesting that more abilities may be retained for longer than may initially appear to be the case from the 'outside'. Henderson comments acerbically that "people with Alzheimer's do actually think" and makes a telling distinction between being able to take part in a conversation and being able to talk if given sufficient time: even when he finds "conversing" difficult, "damn it, still I can talk."[47] He is well aware that he repeats himself incessantly but "we don't want to keep our mouths shut all the time. We want to help."[48] In his diary, he also highlights continuing sources of considerable pleasure, such as music, picking up

41 Fact-finding meeting with members of the Bradford Dementia Group, 29 June 2008; see also Blackman T, Mitchell L, Burton E *et al.* (2003) The accessibility of public spaces for people with dementia; a new priority for the 'open city' *Disability & Society* **18(3)**: 357–71 for a discussion of the social model of disability applied to dementia.

42 See, for example, the interviews with people with moderate to severe dementia described in: Sabat SR (2001) *The Experience of Alzheimer's Disease: Life through a tangled veil* (Oxford: Blackwell).

43 Alzheimer's Association (2008) *Voices of Alzheimer's Disease* (Chicago: Alzheimer's Association).

44 JDI Mutual Support Group (2008) *In the Mists of Memory: A celebration of the circle of life* (Falkirk: JDI); Alzheimer Scotland (2003) *Don't Make the Journey Alone* (Edinburgh: Alzheimer Scotland).

45 Alzheimer's Association (2008) *Voices of Alzheimer's Disease* (Chicago: Alzheimer's Association), p11.

46 *Ibid*, p3.

47 Henderson CS (1998) *Partial View: An Alzheimer's journal* (Dallas: Southern Methodist University Press), pp3, 18 and 21.

48 *Ibid*, p86.

leaves and watching birds,[49] and comments: "we do have feelings and we do have some kind of knowledge."[50]

1.17 We will return, in later Chapters of this Report, to this idea that it is crucial to 'see the person, not only the dementia'[51] and to recognise the dangers of seeing dementia (and by implication those living with dementia) primarily as a collection of negative attributes. At the same time, however, it is important not to minimise the powerful effect that the symptoms and diagnosis of dementia have on those with the condition and on their families and friends.

1.18 Those responding to the Nuffield Council's consultation paper on dementia provided the Working Party with a compelling body of evidence in this respect.[52] Almost half of the 200 respondents had direct family experience of caring for someone with dementia; seven individual respondents themselves had a diagnosis of dementia; and many of the group responses such as those from the Alzheimer's Society, Alzheimer Scotland and local support groups were based on the contributions and insights of people with dementia and carers. Many in their responses expressed concerns about actual or potential loss: loss of mental ability and easy communication, loss of confidence and self-esteem, loss of independence and control over one's own life, and loss of dignity. Strongly associated with this sense of loss came fear of social embarrassment, anxiety about being a burden, especially in the future, and a sense of vulnerability. A third key theme in the responses was the emotional impact of dementia: the anxiety, frustration, depression and changed behaviours associated with the condition. The impact of dementia should never be under-estimated, even while emphasising the importance of focusing on what *can* be achieved.

Social and cultural factors affecting the experience of dementia

1.19 Dementia affects people from all communities and backgrounds. People with dementia have the same basic human needs – for example for comfort, attachment and inclusion – irrespective of their background. However, the *way* these needs show themselves and can be met may depend to a large degree on the person's cultural and social background.[53] Factors associated with ethnicity, for example, such as family and community structures, concepts of family duty, and attitudes and beliefs about old age in general and dementia in particular, are likely to play a significant role in a person's experience of dementia, on the level of disability it creates and on the kind of support required.[54]

1.20 However, socio-economic factors such as income, occupation and education will also play an important role in a person's experience of dementia, and it has been suggested that a focus on culture and ethnicity in isolation may promote misunderstandings and make it harder to provide support that is genuinely appropriate for the individual.[55] In addition to the importance of socio-economic variations within communities, there is also a growing awareness of the extent to which

---

[49] *Ibid*, pp17 and 77.

[50] *Ibid*, p56.

[51] Adapted from Kitwood T (1997) *Dementia Reconsidered: The person comes first* (Buckingham, UK: Open University Press), p7.

[52] Nuffield Council on Bioethics (2008) *Dementia: Ethical issues – consultation paper* (London: Nuffield Council on Bioethics); Nuffield Council on Bioethics (2009) *Dementia: Ethical issues – summary of public consultation* (London: Nuffield Council on Bioethics).

[53] See, for example, Mortimer J (2002) *A Toolkit for Working with Cultural Diversity* (London: Alzheimer's Society); Dementia Plus (2001) *Twice a Child: Dementia care for African-Caribbean and Asian older people in Wolverhampton* (Wolverhampton: Dementia Plus).

[54] See, for example, La Fontaine J, Ahuja J, Bradbury NM, Phillips S and Oyebode JR (2007) Understanding dementia amongst people in minority ethnic and cultural groups *Journal of Advanced Nursing* 60: 605–14; Bowes A and Wilkinson H (2003) 'We didn't know it would get that bad': South Asian experiences of dementia and the service response *Health and Social Care in the Community* 11(5): 387–96; Mackenzie J (2006) Stigma and dementia: East European and South Asian family carers negotiating stigma in the UK *Dementia* 5: 233–47; Iliffe S and Manthorpe J (2004) The debate on ethnicity and dementia: from category fallacy to person-centred care? *Aging & Mental Health* 8(4): 283–92.

[55] Iliffe S and Manthorpe J (2004) The debate on ethnicity and dementia: from category fallacy to person-centred care? *Aging & Mental Health* 8(4): 283–92.

members of the same ethnic community may have very different experiences and expectations, particularly between different generations.[56] Cultural sensitivity will therefore best be achieved by care providers being alert to the beliefs, preferences and experiences of each of those for whom they care, without prior assumptions.[57] This clearly has major educational implications given the wide range of cultures and backgrounds of those both providing and receiving care.

1.21 More individualised factors, such as the individual's personal coping mechanisms when facing adversity, or the existence (or absence) of family support or other informal supportive network, may also play a significant part in how any particular individual experiences and copes with the symptoms of dementia.[58] As we will discuss in Chapter 4, the attitudes of others – the extent to which they are able to accept the person with dementia and adjust their own behaviour appropriately – are also crucial.

The economic impact of dementia

1.22 In addition to its personal and social impact, dementia also has significant financial implications for those with dementia, their families and carers and for the health care and social care systems. In the UK the overall annual economic cost of late-onset dementia was estimated in 2007 at over £17 billion. This figure includes costs resulting from care provided by formal agencies and also the estimated financial value of unpaid care provided by family and friends, with the latter amounting to more than a third of the total.[59] Families and individuals further contribute to the cost of care home accommodation: the National Audit Office notes that 30 per cent of care home fees in England are met in this way, with the result that families bear around half the total cost.[60] The cost in the UK of NHS and local authority social care services provided for people with dementia are estimated at £1.36 billion and £2.5 billion respectively.[61] These dwarf the amounts currently spent on medicines: it is estimated that approximately £82 million was spent on drugs for treating cognitive symptoms in dementia (cholinesterase inhibitors and memantine) in England in 2007.[62]

Scientific understandings of dementia and current research targets

1.23 While there is a growing understanding of the physical changes in the brain associated with the development of the various forms of dementia, the causal mechanisms that result in a person's developing the signs and symptoms of dementia are still far from clear. A number of the dementias are believed to be caused by the accumulation in the brain of a normal protein which becomes abnormally folded and then forms aggregates either outside or inside the nerve cells (neurones).

---

[56] Jutlla K and Moreland N (2007) *The personalisation of dementia services and existential realities: understanding Sikh carers caring for an older person with dementia in Wolverhampton*, paper delivered at the UK Dementia Congress, 6–7 Nov 2007; Seabrooke V and Milne A (2004) *Culture and Care in Dementia: A study of the Asian community in North West Kent* (Northfleet, Kent: Alzheimer's and Dementia Support Services).

[57] Iliffe S and Manthorpe J (2004) The debate on ethnicity and dementia: from category fallacy to person-centred care? *Aging & Mental Health* **8(4)**: 283–92.

[58] Aminzadeh F, Byszewski A, Molnar FJ and Eisner M (2007) Emotional impact of dementia diagnosis: exploring persons with dementia and caregivers' perspectives *Aging & Mental Health* **11(3)**: 281–90; Clare L, Roth I and Pratt R (2005) Perceptions of change over time in early-stage Alzheimer's disease: implications for understanding awareness and coping style *Dementia* **4(4)**: 487–520; Katsuno T (2005) Dementia from the inside: how people with early-stage dementia evaluate their quality of life *Aging & Society* **25**: 197–214.

[59] Knapp M and Prince M (King's College London and London School of Economics) (2007) *Dementia UK* (London: Alzheimer's Society), pxviii; informal care was costed by reference to the cost of a home care worker and to the minimum wage, depending on the tasks performed, and the overall figure includes lost income where carers have given up paid work, but not the value of welfare benefits.

[60] National Audit Office (2007) *Improving Services and Support for People with Dementia* (London: The Stationery Office), p18.

[61] Knapp M and Prince M (King's College London and London School of Economics) (2007) *Dementia UK* (London: Alzheimer's Society), pxviii.

[62] House of Commons *Hansard*, 25 November 2008, cc1214–5W, available at: www.publications.parliament.uk/pa/cm200708/cmhansrd/cm081125/text/81125w0011.htm#08112617000678. Figures relate to the drugs listed in section 4.11 of the British National Formulary.

In Alzheimer's disease, the protein beta-amyloid (Aß) accumulates around the neurones to form 'plaques' and the protein tau accumulates within the neurones to form 'tangles'. In dementia with Lewy bodies, the 'Lewy bodies' are accumulations of alpha-synuclein protein. These and other misfolded proteins are thought to damage neurones in particular functional pathways in the brain, with some structures being more affected than others depending on the particular disease. In vascular dementia, on the other hand, the damage to the neurones is fundamentally caused by the reduced energy supplied to the cells. This can be by direct damage caused by interruption to the blood supply by stroke, or more subtle changes caused by hypertension, and even changes in vessel walls caused by accumulations of amyloid. In other dementias such as frontotemporal dementia, neurones are damaged by the accumulation of the proteins ubiquitin and TDP-43, and also by reductions in the protein progranulin, which would normally help cell growth.

1.24 When neurones are stressed or dying, levels of neurotransmitters (chemical 'messengers' in the brain) are reduced or become less effective. Much of the clinical trial work under way at present has been aimed at identifying drugs that will alter neurotransmitter levels in the damaged pathways and hence provide improvements in the person's cognitive skills and ability to function independently. Some of this research is now translating into treatments. In Alzheimer's disease, for example, cholinesterase inhibitors, which prevent the enzyme acetylcholinesterase from breaking down acetylcholine in the brain, have been by far the most successful drug treatments developed so far. Memantine, which blocks the receptor of the neurotransmitter glutamate, has also shown convincing evidence of efficacy and possibly disease modification.[63]

1.25 Considerable research effort is directed towards 'anti-amyloid' strategies for treating Alzheimer's disease, focusing directly on the role played by the protein beta-amyloid in damaging the neurones. These include attempts to prevent the production of excess amyloid and its subsequent aggregation into plaques;[64] stimulation of the body's own immune system to remove the amyloid;[65] and 'passive' immunisation in which antibodies against amyloid that have been made in the laboratory are used to remove the amyloid.[66] Other areas of investigation include research into the role that inflammation may play in driving or exacerbating the disease process,[67] and the use of nerve growth factor to protect and even restore the 'circuits' within the brain.[68] Strategies trying to alter the processing of the tau protein to prevent the formation of tangles, or to support molecular pathways that generate the energy supply of neurones, are also under way.[69] It is hoped that this will reduce the damaging effects of degeneration on cell function and help maintain normal communication between neurones.

1.26 However, while there is a great deal of enthusiasm for the hypotheses underlying these approaches, research is not, as yet, leading to significant clinical improvements. One explanation for this is the possibility that disease-modifying therapies may work only in the very early stages of dementia, before extensive brain damage has already been caused, and it is not currently possible to identify

---

63 Salloway S, Mintzer J, Weiner MF and Cummings JL (2008) Disease-modifying therapies in Alzheimer's disease *Alzheimer's & Dementia* **4(2)**: 65–79.

64 *Ibid.*

65 Holmes C, Boche D, Wilkinson D *et al.* (2008) Long-term effects of Aß42 immunisation in Alzheimer's disease: follow-up of a randomised, placebo-controlled phase I trial *The Lancet* **372(9634)**: 216–23.

66 Brody DL and Holtzman DM (2008) Active and passive immunotherapy for neurodegenerative disorders *Annual Review of Neuroscience* **31**: 175–93.

67 Perry VH, Cunningham C and Holmes C (2007) Systemic infections and inflammation affect chronic neurodegeneration *Nature Reviews Immunology* **7(2)**: 161–7.

68 Nagahara AH, Merrill DA, Coppola G *et al.* (2009) Neuroprotective effects of brain-derived neurotrophic factor in rodent and primate models of Alzheimer's disease *Nature Medicine* **15(3)**: 331–7.

69 Wischik CM, Bentham P, Wischik DJ and Seng KM (2008) Tau aggregation inhibitor (TAI) therapy with rember™ arrests disease progression in mild and moderate Alzheimer's disease over 50 weeks *Alzheimer's & Dementia* **4(4) (Supplement)**: T167.

people at this stage to participate in the trials.[70] Other difficulties involve the extent to which the mouse models used in research are directly applicable to humans, and the possibility that clinical trials will need to extend over a much longer period than at present in order to identify clinical effects on a person's memory or behaviour.[71]

1.27 As yet, the work on non-Alzheimer's dementias is not as advanced as that on Alzheimer's disease. Similar approaches, however, such as the use of antibodies, are now being considered for other forms of dementia where abnormal protein accumulation is responsible for decline in cell function and cell death.

1.28 While research to modify the effects of dementia or even provide a 'cure' is continuing, it is clearly also important to explore avenues that might prevent the diseases that lead to dementia. Epidemiological studies suggest that risk factors associated with cardiovascular disease may also be risk factors for developing dementia, and strategies aimed at improving exercise and reducing risks such as hypertension and high blood cholesterol have been proposed. The idea that looking after the heart will look after the brain is therefore an attractive one and may influence the future prevalence not only of vascular dementia but also of Alzheimer's disease. Other theories suggest that social activity and engagement may reduce the risk of developing dementia,[72] while cognitive activity in middle age may help develop and maintain a 'cognitive reserve' which may delay the onset of dementia symptoms.[73]

1.29 However, what is not yet clear is whether, once Alzheimer's disease is established, reducing the vascular risk factors will have a significant effect on disease progression. Indeed, the relative importance of these risk factors for Alzheimer's disease remains uncertain.[74] It is also important to note that, if people live longer as a result of living a healthier lifestyle, their risk of developing dementia at the very end of their (extended) life is also likely to increase. Strategies that aim to delay the onset of dementia may therefore not succeed in reducing the total number of people developing dementia before their death, although they may decrease the total amount of time in which the disabling effects of dementia are experienced.[75]

1.30 As our understanding of the physical changes in the brain, both those associated with various forms of dementia and those associated with ordinary ageing, increases, the idea of what a 'cure' for dementia might look like may need to be reconsidered. One idea that has been put forward is that Alzheimer's disease is simply 'accelerated ageing': that is, that everyone, were they to live long enough, would ultimately experience the cognitive decline associated with Alzheimer's. This has been strongly contested: although cognitive abilities do decline in old age and it is difficult to draw a clear line between cognitive losses associated with dementia and those associated with old age, epidemiological studies of the very old suggest that it is not the case that everyone would get Alzheimer's disease were they to live long enough.[76] Moreover, it is well accepted that different

---

[70] Abbott A (2008) The plaque plan *Nature* **456**: 161–4.

[71] *Ibid*; Schnabel J (2008) Standard Model *Nature* **454**: 682–5

[72] Wang H-X, Karp A, Herlitz A *et al.* (2009) Personality and lifestyle in relation to dementia incidence *Neurology* **72**: 253–9.

[73] Carlson MC, Helms MJ, Steffens DC *et al.* (2008) Midlife activity predicts risk of dementia in older male twin pairs *Alzheimer's & Dementia* **4(5)**: 324–31.

[74] Purnell C, Gao S, Callahan CM and Hendrie HC (2009) Cardiovascular risk factors and incident Alzheimer disease: a systematic review of the literature *Alzheimer Disease & Associated Disorders* **23(1)**: 1–10; Yip AG, Brayne C and Matthews FE (2006) Risk factors for incident dementia in England and Wales: The Medical Research Council Cognitive Function and Ageing Study. A population-based nested case-control study *Age and Ageing* **35**: 154–60.

[75] Brayne C, Gao Lu, Dewey M and Matthews FE (2006) Dementia before death in ageing societies: the promise of prevention and the reality *PLoS Medicine* **3(10) e397**; Jagger C, Matthews R, Lindesay J *et al.* (2009) The effect of dementia trends and treatments on longevity and disability: a simulation model based on the MRC Cognitive Function and Ageing Study (MRC CFAS) *Age and Ageing* **38(3)**: 319–25.

[76] See, for example, Anderson E (2008) Cognitive change in old age, in *Oxford Textbook of Old Age Psychiatry*, Jacoby R, Oppenheimer C, Dening T and Thomas A (Editors) (Oxford: Oxford University Press), pp33–50 at p34.

forms of dementia have different causes, and there seems no reason to conflate Alzheimer's disease with ordinary ageing when a different explanation is accepted for other dementias.[77] Nevertheless, the degree of cognitive decline which undoubtedly accompanies old age does challenge the idea that a 'cure' for dementia could ever restore a person's brain to how it was when the person was much younger. A more realistic concept of what a 'cure' for dementia might look like would therefore be action to stop the disease process in its tracks at the point of diagnosis.

1.31 Given that there is little immediate prospect of such a cure being developed,[78] and that those medicines that are currently licensed to slow disease progression have a relatively limited and temporary effect, the importance of maximising the quality of life of those who currently have dementia becomes all the more imperative. More interest is gradually being shown in approaches which focus on treating the way people with dementia feel, and attempting to maximise their independence and quality of life, rather than on seeking a radical 'cure'. There is a growing acceptance that it may be more productive when assessing the benefits of treatment to look at the effect the treatment has had on reducing the person's rate of decline, minimising their level of disability or improving their quality of life, rather than looking for improvement in the way the person scores in a cognitive test.[79] Such an approach could potentially affect both how existing therapies are evaluated and the choice of future areas of research.

1.32 Developments in scientific understandings of the physical mechanisms which underlie many of the symptoms of dementia are also potentially highly valuable in improving the quality of care and support for people with dementia, even where they do not lead directly to disease-modifying therapies. Much distress, for example, may be caused by disinhibited behaviour on the part of a person with dementia, with those close to the person seeing such uncharacteristic behaviour as an example of fundamental personality change. Growing understanding of how such behaviour is linked with damage to the mechanisms in the brain that usually enable people to keep particular thoughts and emotions private will encourage more appropriate responses to such behaviour and help reduce the stress placed on carers.[80]

Diagnosing dementia

Methods of diagnosis

> **Box 1.5: NICE guideline on diagnosis**
>
> A diagnosis of dementia should only be made after a comprehensive assessment, which will include taking the person's medical history, examining their cognitive and mental state, conducting a physical examination, and reviewing their existing medication. Account should be taken of wider factors that may affect a person's performance in cognitive and functional tests, such as any existing physical or mental illnesses or disabilities, their educational level and their former levels of attainment and functioning. Where the diagnosis is mild or questionable, formal neuropsychological testing should be conducted.
>
> Structural imaging should be used to exclude other possible causes of the person's symptoms, and to help establish the subtype of dementia: magnetic resonance imaging (MRI) is preferred but computed tomography (CT) scanning may also be used. Various forms of SPECT (single-photon emission computed tomography) may be used to help differentiate Alzheimer's disease, vascular dementia and frontotemporal dementia, and to help confirm suspected dementia with Lewy bodies. If the person with suspected dementia also has learning disabilities, specialist advice should be sought when interpreting the scans.
>
> NICE/SCIE (2006) *Dementia: Supporting people with dementia and their carers in health and social care,* NICE Clinical Guideline 42 (London: NICE and SCIE).

---

[77]   *Ibid.*

[78]   See, for example, the discussion in paragraph 1.26 and the disappointing results of the immunisation study, where removal of amyloid did not lead to improvements in symptoms: Holmes C, Boche D, Wilkinson D *et al.* (2008) Long-term effects of Aß42 immunisation in Alzheimer's disease: follow-up of a randomised, placebo-controlled phase I trial *The Lancet* **372(9634)**: 216–23.

[79]   Wilkinson D and Andersen HF (2007) Analysis of the effect of memantine in reducing the worsening of clinical symptoms in patients with moderate to severe Alzheimer's disease *Dementia and Geriatric Cognitive Disorders* **24(2)**: 138–45.

[80]   Shulman KI (1997) Disinhibition syndromes, secondary mania and bipolar disorder in old age *Journal of Affective Disorders* **46(3)**: 175–82.

1.33 Other than in specialist research centres, the most accurate diagnosis that can be achieved at present is through a clinical evaluation and diagnosis by an experienced clinician. Routine investigations and a brain scan are also used to exclude any contributory causes of the person's symptoms, such as those due to physical illness or other brain disease, like stroke or tumour. Examination of amyloid and tau in the cerebrospinal fluid (CSF) is thought to increase diagnostic accuracy in early cases of Alzheimer's disease, but is not routinely available outside research centres.[81] New imaging techniques that enable beta-amyloid to be seen on brain scans and hence potentially increase diagnostic accuracy are being developed,[82] but these are not yet available in general clinical practice. Moreover, it is not yet known how well these scans or CSF tests will work in larger older populations, and hence how useful they will be as an accurate diagnostic tool: a major post-mortem study has found a high frequency of individuals showing significant signs of amyloid deposits, which would have appeared as 'positive scans', regardless of whether the person in fact experienced any signs of dementia during their life-time.[83]

> **Box 1.6: Biomarkers**
>
> Biological markers or 'biomarkers' are molecules or sets of different molecules that, when detected at a particular level in body fluids or tissues, indicate the presence of a disease. Biomarkers being developed in dementia include examination of the levels of beta-amyloid or tau proteins in a person's CSF, and the use of a radioactive ligand (a molecule which binds to a protein, in this case beta-amyloid) to make the beta-amyloid visible on a brain scan.

1.34 The clinical diagnosis is based on the history and type of cognitive impairment and its effect on the person's everyday life, combined with corroborative history from someone who knows the person with suspected dementia well. The cognitive impairments are then confirmed through testing with validated procedures, of which the best known is the 'Mini-Mental State Examination' (MMSE) (see paragraph 1.12). The MMSE will then usually be followed by more detailed tests. It is clearly important that people who are beginning to experience possible symptoms of dementia have ready access to experienced teams who are well placed to exclude other possible causes of disorientation or memory loss.

1.35 The accuracy of diagnosis, and whether it will in the future become possible to identify people at risk in the very early stages of the disease, is clearly a key research question. The development of reliable 'biomarkers' could potentially be valuable for a number of purposes: predicting who may, or may not, be likely to develop a particular disease; distinguishing between different types or sub-types of dementia; and acting as a surrogate measure for the effectiveness of medicines both in clinical trials and in clinical practice. There are several promising approaches in the development of biomarkers, at least in the case of Alzheimer's disease, including the new imaging techniques and CSF tests described above (see paragraph 1.33 and Box 1.6). However, these tests are invasive, and while at present they may increase diagnostic certainty, they do not necessarily correlate directly with treatment effects. Clearly a blood or urine test, which would be much less invasive than the lumbar puncture required to obtain CSF, would be useful in developing this work further. As yet, however, no such test is available and the CSF markers have largely been used in people with confirmed disease, and in a limited number of individuals. It is therefore not known whether

---

81 Sonnen JA, Montine KS, Quinn JF *et al*. (2008) Biomarkers for cognitive impairment and dementia in elderly people *The Lancet Neurology* **7(8)**: 704–14.

82 de Leon MJ, Mosconi L, Blennow K *et al*. (2007) Imaging and CSF studies in the preclinical diagnosis of Alzheimer's disease *Annals of the New York Academy of Sciences* **1097**: 114–45.

83 Neuropathology Group of the Medical Research Council Cognitive Function and Ageing Study (2001) Pathological correlates of late-onset dementia in a multicentre, community-based population in England and Wales *The Lancet* **357**: 169–75. See also Savva GM, Wharton SB, Ince PG *et al*. (2009) Age, neuropathology, and dementia *New England Journal of Medicine* **360**: 2302–9, reporting evidence that the strength of the association between the pathological features of Alzheimer's disease and the symptoms of dementia diminishes after age 75.

they will act as useful predictors of disease in all individuals or in the most elderly, who are likely to have complex multiple health problems.[84]

Pre-symptomatic diagnosis and screening

1.36 Given that there is currently neither an effective way of diagnosing the changes in the brain that precede dementia, nor effective treatment to prevent the development of dementia if identified at this early stage, population screening would not be valuable at present.[85] While considerable research effort is being devoted to identifying genetic predispositions to various forms of dementia (for example the ApoE4 gene variant which indicates susceptibility for late-onset Alzheimer's disease) this information cannot yet be used in any useful way for prediction or screening, as the presence of the gene indicates only a relatively small increased risk of developing the condition: many other factors will come into play to determine whether the person in fact goes on to develop the disease.

Ethical questions arising out of this Chapter

1.37 Dementia gives rise to many ethical questions affecting both the individuals directly involved – the person with dementia themselves together with their close family and friends who provide much of their support – and society as a whole. We now know much more about the damage to the brain that leads to the symptoms and behaviours of dementia, but we also have a growing awareness of the abilities and emotions which are retained long into dementia, despite serious cognitive losses. This increased understanding poses a strong challenge to past ideas of dementia as a 'death that leaves the body behind' and raises important questions as to the way in which people with dementia are currently regarded and respected. Yet this increase in knowledge has not yet delivered treatments which have more than a temporary effect. This lack of a 'quick-fix' solution challenges us to look more closely at how people can be supported to live well with dementia, how their experience of disability can be minimised, and the implications of this for both services and research.

1.38 Even with the best support, a person with dementia will experience profound effects in their life as a result of their disease. The decline in mental capacity and ability to function independently, together with the effect dementia may have on mood and behaviour, is highly distressing to the person with dementia themselves, and creates difficulties for carers as they seek to respond appropriately. The potential for frequent and serious conflicts of interest between the person being cared for and their carer or carers generates further ethical difficulties. The increasing number of people developing dementia means that many more people will be facing these questions in their own lives. This raises further ethical questions about how society supports people with dementia, and how it prioritises various forms of research into dementia.

---

[84] de Leon MJ, Mosconi L, Blennow K *et al.* (2007) Imaging and CSF studies in the preclinical diagnosis of Alzheimer's disease *Annals of the New York Academy of Sciences* **1097**: 114–45; Sonnen JA, Montine KS, Quinn JF *et al.* (2008) Biomarkers for cognitive impairment and dementia in elderly people *The Lancet Neurology* **7(8)**: 704–14.

[85] Brayne C, Fox C and Boustani M (2007) Dementia screening in primary care: is it time? *The Journal of the American Medical Association* **298(20)**: 2409–11.

Chapter 2

An ethical framework

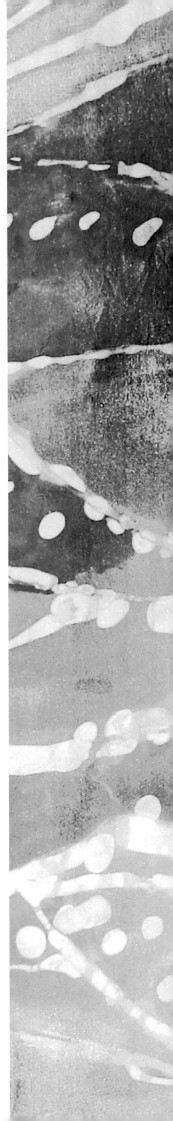

Chapter 2 – An ethical framework

Introduction

2.1   This Report focuses primarily on those ethical issues that are faced by people with dementia themselves and by those directly involved in caring for them. Ethical issues arise, however, for all of us. This is because we all face the possibility of dementia ourselves, and because as members of society we are involved in questions about attitudes towards dementia and about how best those with dementia and their carers should be supported.

2.2   Ethics is concerned with questions about the morally right thing to do. In many situations it may be clear what it is right to do. In other situations, however, there may be several options, none of which is unambiguously right. Such situations create an ethical dilemma for the person making the decision. Different ethical values may point to different courses of action, and deciding on which course to take involves judgment in deciding how much weight to give to each value. There are many examples in this Report of problematic situations that pose ethical difficulties for those involved in the care of people with dementia.

2.3   In ordinary conversation, people often think of ethical issues primarily in terms of 'large' issues, such as end of life decisions, or in connection with sexual behaviour. In this Report the ethical discussions are not limited to these larger issues. Indeed the view taken in this Report is that ethical questions arise very frequently in the ordinary day-to-day care of people with dementia. Carers (families, friends and neighbours providing unpaid care) are making ethical decisions almost every day: how to balance safety with freedom; deciding what is in the best interests of the person with dementia; and balancing the needs of the person with dementia with those of others, including the carers themselves. Care workers and professionals working with people with dementia face similar challenges.

2.4   Ethical issues, whether faced by carers, care workers, professionals or society, arise in specific situations, and the relevant ethical judgments must be made in the light of each particular situation. Ethical judgments should not be arbitrary: they should be based on general values, and those values need to be applied to the specific situation. It is rarely possible, however, simply to deduce from general values the (ethically) right thing to do in each specific situation: ethical judgments are too complex and uncertain. It is, nevertheless, important to provide some structure – an ethical framework – if ethical judgments are to be based on a sound foundation. In this Chapter we propose an ethical framework to help those who face ethical problems in the context of dementia. We explain the framework in considerable detail because the details may help those providing care to make decisions in some of the ethically problematic situations that they face. The framework also underpins the discussions of ethical questions throughout this Report.

The origins of our ethical framework

2.5   The framework that we propose has six components: a methodology for approaching ethical decisions; beliefs about the nature and impact of dementia; and a set of interlinked ethical values. These are listed in Box 2.1 below and explained more fully in the rest of this Chapter.

> **Box 2.1: Dementia: an ethical framework**
>
> **Component 1:** **A 'case-based' approach to ethical decisions:** Ethical decisions can be approached in a three-stage process: identifying the relevant facts; interpreting and applying appropriate ethical values to those facts; and comparing the situation with other similar situations to find ethically relevant similarities or differences.
>
> **Component 2:** **A belief about the nature of dementia:** Dementia arises as a result of a brain disorder, and is harmful to the individual.
>
> **Component 3:** **A belief about quality of life with dementia:** With good care and support, people with dementia can expect to have a good quality of life throughout the course of their illness.
>
> **Component 4:** **The importance of promoting the interests both of the person with dementia and of those who care for them:** People with dementia have interests, both in their autonomy and their well-being. Promoting autonomy involves enabling and fostering relationships that are important to the person, and supporting them in maintaining their sense of self and expressing their values. Autonomy is not simply to be equated with the ability to make rational decisions. A person's well-being includes both their moment-to-moment experiences of contentment or pleasure, and more objective factors such as their level of cognitive functioning. The separate interests of carers must be recognised and promoted.
>
> **Component 5:** **The requirement to act in accordance with solidarity:** The need to recognise the citizenship of people with dementia, and to acknowledge our mutual interdependence and responsibility to support people with dementia, both within families and in society as a whole.
>
> **Component 6:** **Recognising personhood, identity and value:** The person with dementia remains the same, equally valued, person throughout the course of their illness, regardless of the extent of the changes in their cognitive and other functions.

2.6 We have developed our framework in order to respond to the particular dilemmas and difficulties which arise as a result of dementia. The framework draws on existing, widely used approaches to health care ethics. Although there are many different approaches to health care ethics, the value placed on factors such as a person's wishes, values and general well-being, and on broader factors such as some sense of fairness or justice, are common to all.[86] Thus, while our framework is not dependent on any single approach to ethics, it is compatible with other mainstream approaches.

Component 1: A case-based approach to ethical decisions

Sound moral judgments

2.7 Determining the right thing to do in an ethically complicated situation is difficult, and often there is more than one ethically defensible answer to a given question. This is certainly the case for some of the difficult problems presented by dementia and raised by respondents to our consultation. However, we think that 'sound moral judgments' have a number of features, and that a consideration of these features can provide a useful methodology for ethical deliberation.[87] This methodology has three main stages: identifying and clarifying the relevant factual considerations; interpreting and applying appropriate ethical values; and comparing with other similar situations. We describe each of these stages in turn below, and then consider the additional support that those having to make difficult ethical decisions may need in order to cope with the difficulties they face.

Identifying and clarifying relevant factual considerations

2.8 Sound moral judgments are always based upon the careful consideration of the background factors that are relevant to the particular decision. Consider a 70-year-old man, Mr P, living with

---

[86] Respect for autonomy, for example, is highlighted as one of the four key principles in the widely-used text by Beauchamp and Childress (Beauchamp TL and Childress JF (2009) *Principles of Biomedical Ethics*, 6th Edition (New York and Oxford: Oxford University Press)). It is also central in both Kantian and utilitarian approaches to ethics although for very different reasons.

[87] Our account of an approach to sound moral judgments is based upon Jonsen and Toulmin's account of casuistry in Jonsen AR and Toulmin S (1988) *The Abuse of Casuistry: A history of moral reasoning* (Berkeley: University of California Press); Jonsen A (2007) Casuistical reasoning in medical ethics, in *The Principles of Health Care Ethics*, 2nd Edition, Ashcroft R, Dawson A, Draper H and McMillan J (Editors) (Chichester: John Wiley); Jonsen A, Siegler M and Winslade W (1998) *Clinical Ethics* (New York: McGraw-Hill). However, the approach described is not unique to a 'casuistry'-based approach.

his daughter. When his daughter is cooking, Mr P frequently joins her in the kitchen and gets in the way of the cooking. Mr P's daughter is tempted to lock the kitchen door whilst she is cooking to prevent Mr P from entering, but she is not certain whether this is the right thing to do. The relevant facts to consider include: the degree of danger and distress to Mr P when the kitchen door is locked; the length of time he remains distressed after the cooking is finished; the danger if Mr P is in the kitchen; the effect on his daughter of his being in the kitchen during cooking, and the extent to which this interferes with the cooking; what Mr P would have thought about this situation had he considered it before the onset of dementia; and what he is currently able to understand.

Identifying, interpreting and applying relevant ethical values

2.9 Sound moral judgments also involve the consideration of ethical values. For Mr P, general considerations about the importance of autonomy and well-being (see paragraphs 2.26–2.39) need to be interpreted and applied. At first it might seem that concern for Mr P's autonomy would favour allowing him into the kitchen, since locking the door restricts his freedom and his behaviour suggests that he wants to be in the same room as his daughter. This may be too simplistic, however, because Mr P's previous wishes, at a time when he would have understood all the relevant issues, might have favoured enabling his daughter to get on with the cooking unimpeded. Factors affecting Mr P's well-being, such as avoiding harm, also need careful consideration. Finally, the interests of Mr P's daughter are also relevant, both because Mr P's well-being is closely bound up with that of his daughter and because her well-being is of ethical significance in its own right.

Comparison with similar situations

2.10 A third feature of sound moral judgments is they often involve comparison with other similar cases where it has been clear what is the right thing to do ('sentinel' or 'paradigm' cases). When someone faced with a difficult ethical situation has identified the relevant considerations and ethical values, then they can weigh these in the balance and reason on the basis of past experience of similar cases. For example, Mr P's daughter might already have had to make a decision about whether or not to leave her father in the house alone whilst she goes shopping. Her deliberation and conclusions in that situation may be highly relevant to the issue of whether to lock the kitchen door. A health professional such as a community nurse might be able to help the daughter by comparing her situation with that of other families, advising on what has worked elsewhere, and perhaps also by identifying a solution which may remove the problem altogether. In other words, one difficult decision can be compared with another decision where the issue has already been decided. Sometimes this will be easy, if the paradigm case and the present one are very similar; but sometimes there will be both similarities and relevant differences. Yet it might still be helpful to ask: if it is right to lock him in the house when I go shopping, why is it not right to lock him in a part of the house when I am cooking? However, sometimes previous conclusions may have to be revised in the light of new ways of seeing things or new evidence: such a comparison might lead the daughter to decide that it is not right to restrict her father's movements in either of these situations. We return in more detail to quandaries such as these in Chapter 6 (see especially paragraphs 6.28–6.38).

Education and support in ethical decision making

2.11 Legal frameworks and guidelines can often be helpful in guiding practice and decision making, but they need interpreting and applying to specific situations: rarely will a law or guideline provide a sufficiently precise answer to a particular problem, and there are dangers in applying them too rigidly. Some judgment needs to be exercised by those who face these ethical difficulties. Laws and guidelines should support those making decisions, but they should not become a straitjacket and prevent sensible judgment.

2.12 It is therefore not enough, in giving support for the ethical issues that arise for carers, care workers and professionals alike, to provide only guidelines. Skills, as well as knowledge, are required to respond appropriately in these difficult circumstances. If professionals and care workers are to be supported in developing these skills and making decisions about the ethical problems that they face, then they will need both continuing education and forums in which they can discuss and share with others their concerns and approaches. If professionals are to be able to support others, such as carers, in the ethical issues they face, then they will also need ongoing education in how to do this. Crucially, carers will need access to both peer and professional support to enable them to respond to the ethical problems that arise in their lives on a daily basis. We return to the issue of such ongoing education and support in Chapter 7.

Component 2: The nature of dementia

"As with other disabilities [dementia] can be the occasion of positive changes and opportunities, but these should not be romanticised. [...] Dementia is a harm. Nevertheless, while dementia is a form of disability the person with dementia is still a person to whom respect is due." *Professor David A. Jones, consultation respondent*

2.13 Dementia arises as a result of a brain disorder, and people are harmed at some point by having dementia. This statement may seem so obvious as not to need stating but there were some views put to us in the course of our consultation that challenged this belief.[88] For example, it was suggested that if we value the state of having dementia negatively by considering it a disorder, then we are also valuing people who have dementia negatively. It was also argued that with good care people with dementia should be able to have as good a quality of life as people without dementia; and that dementia is on a continuum with normal ageing: that is, the brain degeneration inherent in dementia is within the normal range for brain ageing.

2.14 We reject these three points as grounds for concluding that people are not harmed by having dementia. First, we reject the idea that valuing the state of dementia negatively is the same as valuing the person with dementia negatively. We believe (as we discuss further in paragraph 2.53) that people with dementia should be valued just as much as people without dementia. The state of having dementia is, nevertheless, a harm, and one implication of our position is that if a person could be cured of dementia, or prevented from developing dementia, then in general that would be desirable. By analogy, we can regard the state of having diabetes as a disorder, value it negatively, and aim to prevent and cure diabetes, without in any way valuing people with diabetes themselves in a negative way.

2.15 With regard to the second point, we doubt whether, even with good care, most people with dementia can enjoy as good a quality of life as they enjoyed before they developed dementia. This issue depends on what we understand by 'quality of life'. As we will argue later, a person has interests in the promotion of both their well-being and their autonomy. A person with dementia will not be able to exercise their autonomy to the same extent as prior to the dementia. This represents a harm, regardless of the quality of care the person receives. To deny this would imply that causing brain damage leading to dementia (in a previously healthy person) would not be harmful so long as the person then received good care. Again there is a useful analogy with diabetes. There is a mild state of diabetes where symptoms do not necessarily interfere with having a good quality of life even if the disorder (in the pancreas) is ignored. But at some point the disorder in the pancreas

---

[88] For example, in the Working Party's fact-finding meeting on 29 July 2008, with members of the Bradford Dementia Group.

(like the disorder of the brain in dementia) will intrude and affect the person's life in a harmful way. Good quality care will ameliorate this harm; but this does not contradict the view that the disorder is a harm. Of course none of what we have stated takes away from the importance of providing as good care as possible for people with dementia.

2.16 With regard to the third point, although some neurobiologists consider that dementia is on a spectrum with normal ageing, we take the view that dementia is distinct from ageing (see paragraph 1.30). However, on either view, it is still desirable to prevent or ameliorate its effects. Moreover, we note that the provision of a 'label' for a condition is often the first, and necessary, step for appropriate care and support to be provided.

2.17 There are three key implications of our belief that dementia is a harm:

■ Research into finding ways to prevent or cure dementia, and improve the quality of life of people with dementia, is important, and should be properly resourced (taking into account the prevalence of dementia).

■ Reducing cognitive and other impairments, or slowing the rate of their decline is valuable, although any negative effects associated with such reduction or slowing (such as increased distress on the part of the person about their cognitive abilities) need also to be taken into account.

■ When decisions about resource allocation are made, the dementias should be considered as diseases or illnesses in just the same way as are, for example, the various forms of cancer. Although the question of how society should resource care is beyond the remit of this Report, considerations of justice lead us to conclude that in allocating resources to alleviate the problems that arise as a result of dementia (such as difficulties with self care and the need for support from others in order to achieve a good quality of life), there should be no fundamental difference between those problems and, for example, responding to pain in cancer or mobility difficulties in arthritis. People with dementia should not be disadvantaged by the fact that social care interventions rather than health care are sometimes the appropriate way of helping with the problems that arise as a result of the dementia, nor by the different funding arrangements between social and health care. The need for care, whether social care or health care, is a direct result of the brain disorder.

Component 3: Quality of life in dementia

2.18 Two contradictory approaches to the quality of life people may experience with dementia emerged in the responses to our consultation. One view is that having dementia is so bad that it would be preferable to be dead. Some of those who held this view supported legalising forms of assisted dying for those with dementia who had expressed wishes in advance to that effect. A related position is that it is not a good use of resources for society to put a great deal into the care of people with dementia. It would be better to try to develop laws and practices that facilitate assisted dying, reducing the length of time overall that people live with the condition.

2.19 The contrary view, expressed by many, including those with a great deal of experience caring for people with dementia, was that with good care one can hope, and indeed expect, that people with dementia will have overall a positive quality of life. Some believed that the quality of life with dementia can be just as good as without dementia.

2.20 Without wishing in any way to romanticise dementia, we strongly endorse a version of the second position: that quality of life with dementia can, given proper care, be positive overall for most people, even though the onset of dementia will inevitably lead to the loss or diminution of some valued aspects of a person's life. We note, for example, a research study in the United States of America where 21 out of 23 people with early-stage dementia characterised their current quality of life as 'good' or 'better', despite the fact that most needed some assistance with daily life as a result of their dementia.[89]

2.21 The controversy over this issue is a combination of claims about values and claims about facts. At first sight it might seem that the disagreements relate solely to facts, even if the facts are difficult to determine: that is, is the experience of a person with dementia overall positive or negative? But this is over-simplistic because the experiences of people with dementia vary greatly both between people and at different stages for each person. It is also simplistic because a person's experiences will depend on the care and encouragement they receive, and that care will itself be affected by the views that carers, and society more generally, have towards the possibility of positive experiences.

2.22 More profoundly, those who claim that it would be better to die than to have dementia, do not normally make this claim on the basis of what the actual experience of dementia is like, but rather on the basis of how they *value* certain kinds of experience. In this context it is helpful to distinguish empirical claims about the experiences of people with dementia from value claims. One value claim is that in order for life to be worth living it is necessary not only to be generally happy but also to have a certain level of reflective and deliberative awareness. According to this value judgment, even if a person with dementia is generally happy, perhaps enjoying simple pleasures, such a life is still lacking in value because of the loss of the ability to reflect and deliberate.

2.23 We reject this view for three reasons:

- We believe that a person's life is of value even if they are severely cognitively impaired (see also paragraph 2.53). We do not endorse the view that a life in which a person is cognitively impaired and is experiencing severe behaviour changes is worse than no life at all, even if such developments represent an enormous change from the person's previous functioning. In other words we reject the view that life is worth living only if there is a certain level of reflective and deliberative awareness.

- The question of whether the life of a person with dementia is worse than death depends, in our view, mainly on the nature of the person's day-to-day experiences. This we accept is an area of uncertainty.[90] It is important that further research is carried out to develop methods for determining the quality of these experiences for people with dementia, and we return to this point in Chapter 8. We expect that there is much variation in the quality of these experiences between different people with dementia, and that the experiences will depend crucially on the quality of care. We have been impressed by the evidence of many people and organisations that if skilled support is given to people with dementia and their families, then people with dementia (and their families) can generally have a positive quality of life. Their quality of life is particularly dependent on their relationship with their carers. 'Strange' behaviour, forgetfulness and repetitive questions by the person with dementia may lead to irritation and aggressive responses from carers, and such irritation is likely to be exacerbated if carers fail to understand or accept the changes the person with dementia is experiencing. Quality of life, then, is an issue that is strongly dependent on the relationship between the person with dementia and their carer, and on the carer's understanding of the effects of dementia.

- The view that one takes on this issue is in part about the question of what is worth pursuing. One likely consequence of believing that life with dementia must inevitably be negative is that it is not worthwhile for society to put much effort into improving the lives of people with dementia. This negative valuation might suggest that we should be trying to find ways of ensuring that

---

89 Katsuno T (2005) Dementia from the inside: how people with early-stage dementia evaluate their quality of life *Ageing & Society* **25**: 197–214.

90 See, for example, Edvardsson D, Winblad B and Sandman PO (2008) Person-centred care of people with severe Alzheimer's disease: current status and ways forward *The Lancet Neurology* **7**: 362–7.

people with dementia will soon die. Such a negative valuation is in danger of becoming a self-fulfilling prophecy: the negative valuation leads to indifferent care; indifferent care leads to a poor quality of day-to-day experiences; and the poor quality of experiences provides grounds for the negative valuation. We believe that this approach is wrong. The positive view that we endorse provides an impetus and reasons to try and maximise the positive features, including the quality of day-to-day life, for people with dementia.

Component 4: Promoting interests in autonomy and well-being

2.24 Three sets of interests are of particular importance: the interests of the person with dementia; the interests of carers; and the interests of care workers and professionals. These sets of interests are often closely connected. We will consider first the interests of the person with dementia.

The interests of the person with dementia

2.25 We highlight here two aspects of the interests of the person with dementia: autonomy and well-being.

Autonomy

2.26 Autonomy is often defined as 'self-rule', 'making your own choices', 'ability to live independently' or 'right to self-determination.'[91] Respect for individuals' choices and the promotion of independence are important principles in the care of dependent people, including those with dementia. But what does the right to self-determination mean for people with dementia, particularly when they are highly dependent on the care of others?

2.27 The concept of autonomy is often used to emphasise the freedom to make choices, and 'freedom' may be understood in the sense of 'having no interference' or 'not being hindered by others.' This aspect of autonomy is important in promoting the general right of individuals not to be interfered with against their wishes and provides a basis for the right to information, the right to give or withhold consent to treatment, and the protection of privacy. These are important and enduring moral values in our health care system, and they apply to the care of people with dementia as well as to people with full capacity to make decisions for themselves.

2.28 In the setting of dementia, however, (as in many long-term care settings) this notion of autonomy as 'no interference' is not sufficient. Indeed, if it is not part of a broader notion of autonomy it can be dangerous: it may be interpreted as a 'right to be left alone', degenerating into neglect. Legal norms apparently aimed at promoting autonomy, in this negative sense, can sometimes affect the relationships between professionals and patients, leading practitioners to adopt defensive attitudes and limit their services to care which is immediately necessary or for which patients have given their explicit consent. A person with dementia who walks out of a doctor's consulting room, for example, might be understood as refusing assessment or treatment, while in fact there could be many other reasons for their behaviour. This 'no interference' approach to autonomy may lead to relationships turning into contractual ones defined solely in terms of rights rather than relationships based on caring.

2.29 A further but related problem with some traditional accounts of autonomy is the emphasis on *rationality*: the idea that the ability to exercise autonomy and the ability to make rational decisions are one and the same thing. This can lead to the idea that respect for autonomy is either irrelevant in the context of dementia or that it is related only to what the person wanted before the onset

---

[91] See, for example, the discussion of theories of autonomy in Beauchamp TL and Childress JF (2009) *Principles of Biomedical Ethics*, 6th Edition (New York and Oxford: Oxford University Press), pp100–2.

of dementia. As a result, too little attention is given to the individual's current wishes and feelings which, we believe, are also an expression of their autonomy.

2.30 We believe that these 'negative' and 'rationalistic' accounts of autonomy are not only insufficient in the context of dementia but also problematic. They are problematic because they may promote a negative view of dependence, and "the frail and infirm old who require long-term care are especially vulnerable to the pejorative meanings associated with dependence."[92] The concept of autonomy that we believe is relevant in dementia must give more emphasis to several additional perspectives.

2.31 First, enabling autonomy entails providing active support to the person with dementia so that they can be encouraged to retain and express their sense of self, rather than simply being protected from harm or interference. In order to give this support it is necessary for those providing care to try to understand what the person with dementia is feeling, wanting and experiencing. As a person's dementia becomes more severe, this will become more difficult, but if someone has limited capability to live independently or to realise their own choices, then respect for autonomy must involve others taking active steps to act as advocates and to try to promote their autonomy. Autonomy as freedom from interference completely misses the point that promoting autonomy will often require the provision of active support.

2.32 Secondly, in considering what it means to enhance autonomy, we must recognise that people are not isolated individuals, but are people whose identity is embedded in a network of relationships. A key aspect of who we are is founded on our relationships with those whom we love and others who are important to us. Enabling and promoting autonomy thus involves enabling and fostering relationships that are important to the person. The interests of the person with dementia, including their autonomy interests, are closely linked to the interests of those close to them, and particularly to the interests of their family and friends who are caring for them. This is an important reason why carers should receive advice and support, and this in itself can be helpful to the person with dementia as a way to enhance their autonomy.

2.33 Thirdly, traditional concepts of autonomy emphasise rationality at the expense of emotional factors. This can lead to an approach whereby once a person lacks (rational) capacity to make a particular decision, then respecting autonomy is assumed to relate only to the views held or decisions made by the person before losing capacity. We believe, however, that enhancing the autonomy of a person with dementia includes giving weight to their emotional responses, for example enabling them to pursue activities that they appear to enjoy even if they lack the capacity to make relevant decisions. As we discuss later in the context of personhood (see paragraphs 2.48–2.53), we also believe that people retain the ability to *value* one thing over another even after they have lost the rational ability to formulate and communicate a particular decision.

2.34 Several writers have provided rich accounts of autonomy emphasising and developing these additional perspectives. The terms *relational autonomy* and *actual autonomy* have been used to mark these richer accounts.[93] A key implication of these accounts is that the dependency of people as a result of their disease does not mean that their autonomy cannot be promoted, nor that promoting autonomy simply involves respecting the wishes and values they had before the onset of dementia. On the contrary, it means that people who have become dependent on others through the development of dementia may need support from those who care for them to help them retain their autonomy, and with it their sense of self.

Well-being

2.35 We have argued, on grounds of respecting autonomy, that it is important to pay close attention to the expressed desires and feelings of a person with dementia. Even if our account of autonomy is rejected, however, in favour of an account that sees rationality as so central that a person with moderate or severe dementia would be considered as incapable of expressing autonomous desires, it would still be important to pay close attention to these desires and feelings, and to do everything possible to help the person achieve their desired goals. This is on the grounds of *well-being*. A person with dementia clearly has an interest in being helped to maximise their well-being, an important aspect of which will be related to the satisfaction of their desires and preferences.

2.36 Several different approaches to well-being have been taken by philosophers. In the context of this Report we wish to highlight two approaches that we believe are relevant to people with dementia. The first approach focuses on a person's moment-to-moment experiences. At any one time we experience a certain level of happiness or sadness, of pleasure or pain. Maximising well-being, on this approach, would require maximising the overall sum of positive experiences, where this overall sum is made up of balancing the degrees and duration of positive experiences against the degrees and duration of negative experiences.[94] We believe that this is an important component of well-being and that a person with dementia has a strong interest in having positive experiences such as contentment or pleasure, on a moment-to-moment and day-to-day level.

2.37 The second approach to well-being is what has been called the 'objective list' theory. According to this approach, a person's well-being is not only determined by their overall happiness: it is also affected by things that are objectively good or bad independently of their influence upon happiness.[95] Most objective list theories will include autonomy as something that makes life go well. So on this view, the richer conceptions of autonomy that we have discussed above also contribute to a person's well-being. In the context of dementia, an important example of what contributes to objective well-being, and which is related to autonomy, is a person's level of cognitive dysfunction. It is our view that a person's well-being is negatively affected by such dysfunction, so that reduced cognitive functioning, for example as a result of sedative medication, constitutes a reduction in a person's overall well-being. Equally, a slowing down in a person's deterioration in cognitive functioning (for example owing to treatment) may prevent further deterioration of that person's well-being.

2.38 In considering overall well-being, therefore, both moment-to-moment experiences and cognitive dysfunction are important. A treatment that reduced distress but also increased cognitive impairment would either reduce or increase well-being depending on the balance between the effects, and both effects should be taken into account in coming to a judgment. Similarly, a treatment that reduced the deterioration in cognitive functioning, even if the person remained more distressed because of greater insight into their condition, *might* be justified on the grounds that it contributed to overall well-being. Again our view is that both effects are relevant in coming to a decision, and that the strength of each effect should be closely considered when determining whether or not the treatment would enhance the person's overall well-being.

2.39 One important implication of this is that the moment-to-moment experiences (of pleasure and happiness or pain and unhappiness) are important even if no memory of that moment's experience is retained. Moreover, the level of positive experience is likely to be dependent on the details of

---

[94] See, for example, Griffin J (1986) *Well-being: Its meaning, measurement and moral importance* (Oxford: Clarendon Press).
[95] For an example of an 'objective list' theory see John Finnis (1980) *Natural Law and Human Rights* (Oxford: Oxford University Press).

the person's life and the details of care. This is one reason why in Chapter 3 we will emphasise the importance of paying attention to the details of care and their impact on what the person is experiencing. Indeed, such concern for the ordinary and day-to-day experience is also relevant to autonomy, which can be promoted by enabling the person with dementia to make choices in the apparently small things in life – when to have a cup of tea, for example. Both autonomy and well-being might also be enhanced through enabling people with dementia to engage in productive or meaningful activities. As one of our peer reviewers put it, even "people with profound disabilities are often still able to make simple things which they can appreciate are of value to others."

The interests of carers

2.40 Unpaid carers (family, friends and neighbours) provide most of the care for people with dementia, often motivated and sustained by bonds of love. Their interests are important for two reasons. First, carers are people in their own right, with the same strong claim as people with dementia to have their interests considered. In their role as carers they may face stresses and difficulties, and they may often feel that their own interests have become subordinate to those for whom they provide care. Both professionals and society more generally have duties to try to support carers, both in their caring role and as people with their own independent existence and interests. Secondly, the autonomy and well-being of the person with dementia are closely linked in with their relationships with those close to them (see paragraph 2.32).[96] Support which promotes the interests of carers may also, therefore, act to promote the well-being and autonomy of the person with dementia.

2.41 For both these reasons, support to carers of people with dementia is a crucial part of the services that should be provided in dementia care, and the interests of carers, as individuals, should be considered when difficult ethical decisions involving conflicting interests need to be made.

The interests of professionals and care workers

2.42 A key duty of care workers and professionals is to promote the interests of the person with dementia. This work is demanding and, as with carers, the ability of such professionals and care workers to carry out this work effectively will be enhanced by their receiving proper support themselves. This has implications for the conditions under which they work: the status of, and remuneration for, their work; the work environment, including staffing levels; the way in which they are themselves treated by their employers; and the ongoing education and mentoring that they receive.

Component 5: Solidarity

"...when men and women seem by one consent to open their shut-up hearts freely, and to think of people below them as if they really were fellow-passengers to the grave, and not another race of creatures bound on other journeys." Charles Dickens, *A Christmas Carol*

2.43 Solidarity is the idea that we are all 'fellow-travellers' and that we have duties to support and help each other and in particular those who cannot readily support themselves. Within a society or country solidarity often comes to the fore at times of stress such as war or natural disaster. The high prevalence of dementia, and the fact that we all face a significant risk of developing dementia as we get older, might enable us to develop a particular sense of solidarity with each other in the context of dementia and dementia care.

---

[96] Hughes JC, Hope T, Reader S and Rice D (2002) Dementia and ethics: the views of informal carers *Journal of the Royal Society of Medicine* **95**: 242–6.

2.44 The concept of solidarity underpins the duty of individuals and of society to support those with dementia and their carers. It reinforces the responsibility of all of us to try to help research and to act to de-stigmatise dementia. Solidarity is relevant also to individual relationships: personal solidarity, in the form of love, loyalty and compassion, is the basis and motivation for giving care to one's partner, parent or friend. We suggest, therefore, that, under solidarity, society has a twofold obligation to provide resources and support to people with dementia and their carers: first as part of our obligations to help those who cannot readily support themselves; and secondly to enable carers to maintain their personal solidarity with the person for whom they are caring. Lack of professional support may put carers under extreme pressure. They suffer exhaustion, lacking time or energy for sustaining an affectionate and supportive caring relationship. Likewise, a failure to show solidarity towards care workers, in the form of appropriate support and recognition, can affect their ability to develop and sustain supportive relationships with the people for whom they care.

2.45 When considering the idea of solidarity, those receiving care and support should not be seen simply as people with particular rights or as victims of disease or disability, but rather as citizens with both their own needs and a societal role. People with dementia may need assistance in order to be empowered and given a voice, but they should also be included as citizens with their own views on how solidarity should be practised, and with their own contribution to make.[97]

2.46 Justice, which is at the root of our notion of solidarity, is often defined as a fair distribution of benefits and burdens, particularly in connection with misfortunes for which we cannot be held personally responsible. Given the potential vulnerability of people with dementia, it is particularly important that the allocation of resources results in a supportive environment in dementia care. This is in part an issue of appropriate resources and practical support, but also requires both carers and care workers to be recognised and valued as people who have an important expertise and role in society.

2.47 A fair distribution of benefits and burdens should promote and sustain solidarity, realised as a willingness to support the person with dementia throughout the course of their dementia and to help them in maintaining their autonomy as much as possible.

Component 6: Recognising personhood

2.48 Some philosophers have argued that a person with severe dementia ('person B') may quite literally be a different person – have a different identity – from the person before the dementia ('person A'). This position has its origins in the view that to be able to identify oneself as the same person over time requires memory.[98] There has been considerable philosophical debate over this issue.[99] Some carers also consider the person with dementia as a 'different person' from before, although this is not often meant literally but instead refers to major and distressing changes in mood and behaviour resulting from the dementia.

---

[97] See also: Houtepen R and ter Meulen RHJ (2000) The expectations of solidarity: matters of justice, responsibility and identity in the reconstruction of the health care system *Health Care Analysis* **8**: 355–76.

[98] Locke J (1700) *An Essay Concerning Human Understanding*, Woolhouse R (Editor) (London: Penguin Classics 1997), p302: "since consciousness always accompanies thinking, and 'tis that, that makes every one to be, what he calls self; and thereby distinguishes himself from all other thinking things; in this alone consists *personal identity*, i.e. the sameness of a rational being; and as far as this consciousness can be extended backwards to any past action or thought, so far reaches the identity of that person; it is the same *self* now it was then; and 'tis by the same *self* with this present one that now reflects on it, that that action was done."

[99] See, for example, Buchanan A (1988) Advance directives and the personal identity problem *Philosophy and Public Affairs* **17**: 277–302; Hope T (1994) Personal identity and psychiatric illness, in *Philosophy, Psychology and Psychiatry*, Griffiths AP (Editor) (Cambridge: Cambridge University Press), pp131–43; Dresser R (1995) Dworkin on dementia: elegant theory, questionable policy *Hastings Center Report* **25(6)**: 32–8; Hughes JC, Louw SJ and Sabat SR (Editors) (2006) *Dementia: Mind, meaning, and the person* (Oxford: Oxford University Press).

2.49 The view that a person literally changes identity has profound implications. One implication is that an advance decision made by person A (the person with capacity before the dementia), and person A's values, are irrelevant in making decisions about person B. A second implication is that person A has ceased to exist and this raises the question of what to do with his or her property. A third implication is that the relatives and friends of person A have no long-standing relationship or ties with, and few duties towards, person B. Many philosophers reject this view and argue for the common-sense position that even if the person's mood, behaviour and memory change profoundly, the person with severe dementia is still the same person as before the onset of dementia. According to this latter view, personal identity depends on other (additional) factors, for example on bodily identity,[100] and on interpersonal identity established through relationships with others.[101]

2.50 The various positions on these issues reflect current philosophical controversies which are partly metaphysical in nature. We do not aim to settle these controversies, but simply to offer practical and policy guidance regarding ethical issues arising in the care of people with dementia. From this perspective we believe that the position that a person retains their identity throughout the course of dementia (even though they may behave in profoundly different ways) provides a better guide to policy and practice. The facts of bodily identity, and social connections, in particular, provide important grounds for considering a person as the same person throughout the full course of the illness. Some implications of this position are: that the views and values of the person before the onset of dementia may be relevant in making decisions; that the resources that the person has accumulated during their life may be used for their benefit; and that family and friends may retain responsibilities, and also expectations, that are normally assumed. This position also avoids some of the major practical problems that are associated with the alternative, particularly those associated with considering that one person has died (the person before the onset of severe dementia) and that a new person has come into existence – a person without any social connections. In short, although mood and behaviour may be profoundly affected by dementia, personal identity is not: the individual remains the same person throughout the process of dementia.

2.51 A further view, which we also reject, is that in severe dementia the individual may not merely have a different identity but may cease to be a 'person' at all. This view is based on the idea that in order to be a 'person', a certain level of cognitive functioning is required, and that in severe dementia such cognitive functioning may fall below the required level. The practical implications of this view might include: that the individual with severe dementia should not enjoy the protections of the law that are given to 'persons'; that the individual with dementia does not have any interests, or none beyond those of other (non-human) living creatures; that those close to the individual with dementia no longer have any interests or duties towards them; and perhaps that the views and values of the individual before the onset of dementia are no longer relevant in making decisions about their care.

2.52 This view – that in severe dementia an individual may cease to be a person at all – is subject to as much philosophical controversy, as is the issue of personal identity. There are two principal reasons why we reject this view. The first is uncertainty over what an individual with severe dementia is experiencing, and what is going on in the individual's mind. It has been argued that we should think of people with dementia as 'valuers': people capable of valuing.[102] Most of the time the

---

[100] Matthews E (2006) Dementia and the identity of the person, in *Dementia: Mind, meaning, and the person*, Hughes JC, Louw SJ and Sabat SR (Editors) (Oxford: Oxford University Press), pp163–77.

[101] See, for example, Agich GJ (2003) *Dependence and Autonomy in Old Age: An ethical framework for long-term care* (Cambridge: Cambridge University Press); Kitwood T (1997) *Dementia Reconsidered: The person comes first* (Buckingham, UK: Open University Press), p8.

[102] Jaworska A (1999) Respecting the margins of agency: Alzheimer's patients and the capacity to value *Philosophy and Public Affairs* **28(2)**: 105–38. This point was also endorsed by people with first-hand experience of dementia at the Working Party's fact-finding meeting on 10 July 2008.

person with dementia will be able to convey their values, and the ability to value may persist, even into severe dementia, when the person's inclinations can still be shown by facial features, by gestures and by the expression of emotions.[103] Examples cited by individual Working Party members included powerful responses to music or strong emotional attachments to pets demonstrated by people with severe dementia, even where such attachments had not been particularly important to them in the past.

2.53 Secondly, the view that someone with profound dementia has little value and no interests is based on seeing personhood exclusively in terms of cognitive abilities. However, emotional and spiritual aspects of a person's life are also relevant to personhood, and the various perspectives discussed above in the context of personal identity may also be relevant to personhood itself. Religious approaches to the nature of 'personhood' emphasise the belief that humans do not have to prove their worth as persons, and that it is our capacity to 'be' rather than our capacity to 'do' that gives us value as a person.[104] Such a belief is shared by many non-religious thinkers, who argue for the equality of human worth, regardless of the abilities or merits of any particular individual.[105] If we see people as both situated in a network of relationships and 'embodied' in their own physical presence, then an individual even with severe dementia remains the same, equally valuable, person, throughout the duration of their entire illness.[106]

A note on dignity

2.54 The idea of *human dignity*, and of treating people with *dignity*, is widely used in discussions of ethics and health care, and has been used in many ways, leading some philosophers to consider that it is too vague a concept to be useful.[107] Some, while seeing value in the idea, nevertheless caution that "the concept of human dignity ... is something of a loose cannon ... it can oversimplify complex questions."[108] One analysis of the idea of dignity distinguishes between dignity as a "constraint" and dignity as "empowerment."[109] Dignity may constrain, in the sense that certain actions are absolutely forbidden as being counter to human dignity. Dignity may also empower, by underpinning the ethical importance of treating a person in a way which maintains and upholds their value as a human being.

2.55 We believe that it is the idea of treating a person with dignity, in the sense of 'dignity as empowerment', that can be particularly helpful in the setting of dementia care. In many situations it is immediately apparent what would be meant by treating a person with dignity and what it would mean to treat a person in an undignified manner. For example, it would be wrong, in the setting of a care home, to leave a woman with dementia in the sitting room only partially clothed. It would not be right, in our opinion, to defend such behaviour by saying that the person was unaware that she was only partially dressed and that therefore she was not harmed by it. One way of expressing what is wrong with treating a person in this way is to say that it does not affirm or respect her dignity, that it does not reflect the way those working in the care home would themselves like to be treated. Because there is a general and widespread understanding

[103] Dekkers WJM (2004) Autonomy and the lived body in cases of severe dementia, in *Ethical Foundations of Palliative Care for Alzheimer Disease*, Purtilo RB and ten Have HAMJ (Editors) (Baltimore and London: Johns Hopkins University Press), pp115–30.

[104] See, for example, MacKinlay E (Editor) (2008) *Ageing, Disability and Spirituality: Addressing the challenge of disability in later life* (London and Philadelphia: Jessica Kingsley), pp11–21.

[105] See, for example, Vlastos G (1969) Human worth, merit, and equality, in *Moral Concepts*, Feinberg J (Editor) (London: Oxford University Press), pp141–52.

[106] Aquilina C and Hughes JC (2006) The return of the living dead: agency lost and found?, in *Dementia: Mind, meaning, and the person* Hughes JC, Louw SJ and Sabat SR (Editors) (Oxford: Oxford University Press), pp143–61.

[107] For discussion of this see Ashcroft R (2005) Making sense of dignity *Journal of Medical Ethics* **31**: 679–82.

[108] Beyleveld D and Brownsword R (1998) Human dignity, human rights, and human genetics *Modern Law Review* **61**: 661–81 at 662.

[109] Beyleveld D and Brownsword R (2001) *Human Dignity in Bioethics and Biolaw* (Oxford: Oxford University Press).

of what respects dignity in this sense, it is useful for those caring for people with dementia, and for those involved in setting standards in dementia care, to think about how the dignity of people with dementia can best be respected and what actions and attitudes may undermine it. The concept of dignity is valuable, therefore, in guiding attitudes and approaches to the care of people with dementia. It emphasises the importance of attending to the details of care and a concern for what the person and their relatives might be experiencing.

2.56 The concept of dignity does not stand alone, however, and its importance and value can be derived, we believe, from the ethical framework that we have set out in this Chapter. On the basis of our analysis there are at least three reasons why treating a person in an undignified way may be morally wrong. First, the person might feel uncomfortable or demeaned, even if she cannot express what she wants, or the fact that she is upset. Thus, treating a person in this way may be contrary to the promotion both of her current autonomy and her well-being. Secondly, even if it were true, in the above example, that the person with dementia was unaware of, and unaffected by, the way she is left in the sitting room, this is likely to be against her past autonomy interests – her interests in having the views and values that she had previously held respected. Thirdly, treating a person in this way risks treating her as an 'object' rather than as a person; treating with dignity is a key part of showing respect for the personhood of the individual, recognising her value as a person, equal to anyone without dementia.

Conclusions

2.57 We summarise in Box 2.1 above the six components that we have outlined in this Chapter, and which we believe provide a helpful framework for tackling the ethical problems which arise continually in dementia. In the remaining Chapters of this Report, we will consider how this framework may be of assistance in a number of different areas where ethical difficulties arise: in general approaches to care and support; in the relationships between people with dementia and others in society; when making health and welfare decisions; in aspects of care which pose particular challenges; in the consideration of carers' own interests; and in research.

Chapter 3

What is an ethical approach to care?

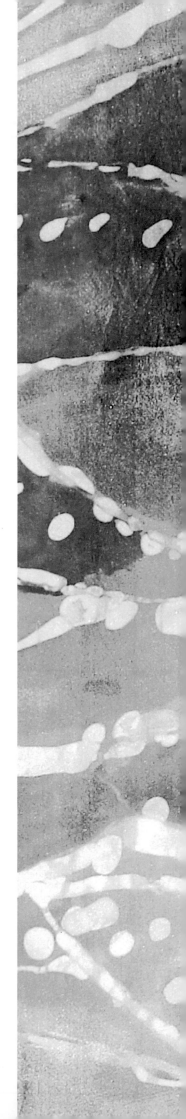

Chapter 3 – What is an ethical approach to care?

Introduction

3.1 In the previous Chapter we put forward a framework to support ethical judgments in the context of dementia, while emphasising that there is rarely one right answer in any given situation. In this Chapter we will discuss how this framework might be practically applied in the day-to-day care of people with dementia, whether in their own homes, or living in some form of supported or residential care. We will then consider in turn various aspects of a 'care pathway' in the light of both our framework and the responses we received to our consultation. The care pathway experienced by any particular individual with dementia will, of course, vary considerably, depending on their own needs and circumstances and the availability of different kinds of support. By looking at scenarios which are likely to arise at various stages of dementia, including assessment and diagnosis, initial advice and support, ongoing support in the community, residential care and palliative care, we seek to suggest ways in which our ethical framework may help those providing care. We illustrate these by reference to services that have come to our notice where aspects of our ethical framework are being realised in practice. In doing this we are also aware that the research base for the relative effectiveness, cost-effectiveness, and transferability of different models of care and support services provided for people with dementia is still relatively limited,[110] and hence it may not always be the case that services that are successful in one area can be readily imitated in another. We return to this issue in Chapter 8 (see paragraphs 8.8 and 8.18).

3.2 Guidance on standards and approaches to the care of people with dementia have recently been the focus of a number of major reports within the UK. In February 2006, SIGN produced a 'clinical guideline', based on a review of the best available evidence, setting out in detail how people with dementia and their carers should be supported by health and social care professionals in Scotland.[111] Later in the same year, NICE and SCIE published a similar guideline for England and Wales.[112] In 2008, the Scottish Government declared dementia a national priority, setting a target of 2011 for all health boards to deliver improvements in early diagnosis and management of people with dementia,[113] and subsequently promising a dementia strategy.[114] In February 2009, the Department of Health in England published a 'National Dementia Strategy', seeking to address three main themes: raising awareness; early diagnosis and intervention; and improving the quality of care.[115] In Wales, a draft National Dementia Action Plan is subject to consultation until September 2009,[116] while in Northern Ireland, the NI Executive has noted the "200 per cent increase in dementia" expected over the next ten years, and promised to work with housing and health authorities to address the needs of people with dementia.[117] We briefly summarise the conclusions of NICE/SCIE guidance, the Scottish

[110] See, for example, Burns A and Robert P (2009) The National Dementia strategy in England *British Medical Journal* **338**: 614 and the research recommendations in SIGN (2006) *Management of Patients with Dementia: A national clinical guideline* (Edinburgh: SIGN), paragraph 6.4.

[111] SIGN (2006) *Management of Patients with Dementia: A national clinical guideline* (Edinburgh: SIGN).

[112] NICE/SCIE (2006) *Dementia: Supporting people with dementia and their carers in health and social care*, NICE Clinical Guideline 42 (London: NICE and SCIE).

[113] NHS Scotland (2008) *Mental Health in Scotland: Dementia – A national priority summary paper* (Edinburgh: The Scottish Government).

[114] Scottish Government news release (2009) Care for dementia, 28 May, available at: www.scotland.gov.uk/News/Releases/2009/05/27152029.

[115] Department of Health (2009) *Living Well with Dementia: A national dementia strategy* (London: Department of Health).

[116] Welsh Assembly Government (2009) *National Dementia Action Plan for Wales*, consultation draft (Cardiff: Department for Health and Social Services).

[117] Northern Ireland Government news release (2008) *Two hundred per cent increase in dementia in next ten years needs addressed says Ritchie*, 31 Jan, available at: www.northernireland.gov.uk/news/news-dsd/news-dsd-january-2008/news-dsd-310108-two-hundred-per-cent.htm.

National Priority Summary Paper, the English National Dementia Strategy and the draft National Dementia Action Plan for Wales (see Boxes 3.1–3.4 below) and, while we broadly endorse their main conclusions and recommendations, we go on to make further observations and recommendations in the light of the ethical framework we have set out.

Box 3.1: NICE/SCIE guidance on health and social care support for people with dementia – key priorities

Non-discrimination: people with dementia should not be excluded from any service because of their diagnosis, age, or co-existing learning disabilities.

Valid consent must be sought from people with dementia. If the person lacks capacity to make a particular decision, then the provisions of the Mental Capacity Act 2005 should be followed.

Carers should receive an assessment of their own needs, and carers experiencing psychological distress should be offered psychological therapy from a specialist.

Health and social care services should be integrated and care plans endorsed by the person with dementia and/or their carers.

Memory assessment services should be the single point of referral for all people with a possible diagnosis of dementia.

Structural imaging (MRI or CT scanning) should be used in the assessment of people with suspected dementia, to exclude other causes of their symptoms and to help establish their specific diagnosis.

People with behaviour that challenges should be offered an early assessment to identify the likely factors that may generate, aggravate or improve the behaviour. Individual care plans should then be developed and regularly reviewed.

Dementia-specific training should be available to all staff working with older people in the health, social care and voluntary sectors.

Acute and general hospitals should plan and provide services that meet the specific needs of people with dementia who need to use hospital services for whatever reason.

NICE/SCIE (2006) *Dementia: Supporting people with dementia and their carers in health and social care*, NICE Clinical Guideline 42 (London: NICE and SCIE).

Box 3.2: Objectives in the Scottish National Priority Summary Paper

- Improvements in early diagnosis and management of people with dementia;
- Improving standards of care through 'integrated care pathways' for dementia;
- Production of information about coping with dementia for people with dementia and for carers;
- Development of appropriate post-diagnostic support services;
- Improving quality of life in hospital and other care settings;
- Improving palliative care;
- Encouragement of 'dementia-friendly' premises;
- Supporting staff, with guidance published on the knowledge, skills and values needed by nurses working with older people's mental health services;
- Raising public awareness; and
- Development of a Scottish Dementia Research Network.

NHS Scotland (2008) *Mental Health in Scotland: Dementia: A national priority summary paper* (Edinburgh: The Scottish Government).

Box 3.3: Objectives in the English National Dementia Strategy

1. Improving public and professional awareness and understanding of dementia;
2. Good-quality early diagnosis and intervention for all;
3. Good-quality information for those with diagnosed dementia and their carers;
4. Enabling easy access to care, support and advice following diagnosis;
5. Development of structured peer support and learning networks;
6. Improved community personal support services;
7. Implementing the Carers' Strategy;
8. Improved quality of care for people with dementia in general hospitals;
9. Improved intermediate care for people with dementia;
10. Considering the potential for housing support, housing-related services and telecare to support people with dementia and their carers;
11. Living well with dementia in care homes;
12. Improved end of life care for people with dementia;
13. An informed and effective workforce for people with dementia;
14. A joint commissioning strategy for dementia;
15. Improved assessment and regulation of health and care services and of how systems are working for people with dementia and their carers;
16. A clear picture of research evidence and needs; and
17. Effective national and regional support for implementation of the Strategy.

Department of Health (2009) *Living Well with Dementia: A national dementia strategy* (London: Department of Health), pp12–3.

> **Box 3.4: Objectives in the draft National Dementia Action Plan for Wales**
>
> **Strengthening individuals:**
>
> ■ Provide good quality information for people with dementia and their carers;
> ■ Acknowledge and support carers as key partners in the care of people with dementia;
> ■ Increase housing options;
> ■ Maximise use of telecare and assistive technology;
> ■ Improve dementia care in the home;
> ■ Provide appropriate end of life care.
>
> **Strengthening communities:**
>
> ■ Increase awareness and understanding;
> ■ Improve the skills of the dementia workforce;
> ■ Improve community crisis intervention;
> ■ Ensure effective joint planning and commissioning.
>
> **Improving infrastructure and access to services for all:**
>
> ■ Ensure timely diagnosis;
> ■ Ensure appropriate use of anti-psychotic medication;
> ■ Ensure appropriate medicines management;
> ■ Improve dementia care in general and community hospitals;
> ■ Improve dementia care in mental health hospitals;
> ■ Improve continuing health care;
> ■ Improve access to intermediate care.
>
> **Making structural changes to economic, cultural and environmental conditions:**
>
> ■ Promote healthy living initiatives in dementia;
> ■ Promote dementia research;
> ■ Take action to ensure the National Plan is implemented.
>
> Welsh Assembly Government (2009) *National Dementia Action Plan for Wales*, consultation draft (Cardiff: Department for Health and Social Services), pp9–11.

Some general points about the care of people with dementia

"If you really want to help somebody, first of all you must find him where he is and start there. This is the secret of caring." [118]

3.3 We argued in Chapter 2 that while dementia is a disorder that is harmful, nevertheless a good quality of life is possible with dementia if the person with dementia is seen and respected as a person with values and interests towards whom we have the same duties as any other fellow human beings. We have also suggested that amongst the key values underpinning our approach to dementia should be concern for the autonomy and well-being of the person with dementia, coupled with an attitude of solidarity based on the belief that we are all 'fellow-travellers' and dependent, to various degrees at different times in our lives, on each other. How can these values be translated into practice on a day-to-day basis in a care environment?

3.4 It will not always be possible to provide services, or support individuals, in a way which fully respects all these values. Some degree of compromise between maximising autonomy and well-being may sometimes be necessary, for example when a person would be at significant risk of harm if they were not restrained in some way. Balancing the interests of the person with dementia with the interests of carers is also sometimes necessary. In many cases the role of support will be central in how the balances and compromises are managed. For example, as the diagram below shows,[119] the participants in our public deliberative event tackled ethical problems by starting with an 'ideal' position of what the person most wanted and valued; then they considered what risks this posed (both to the person with dementia and others); and finally they put forward suggestions of support

---

[118] Kierkegaard S (1998) The point of view, in *Kierkegaard's Writings Volume XXII* (Princeton: Princeton University Press), part 2, chapter 1A, paragraph 2.

[119] Adapted from Opinion Leader (2008) *Deliberative Workshop on Dementia: A report prepared for the Nuffield Council on Bioethics* (London: Opinion Leader), p16.

or adaptations which could maximise the ideal position with minimum risk. In doing so, they demonstrated clearly that it was possible to come to a conclusion that recognised the importance of the various values, without prioritising one at the expense of another.

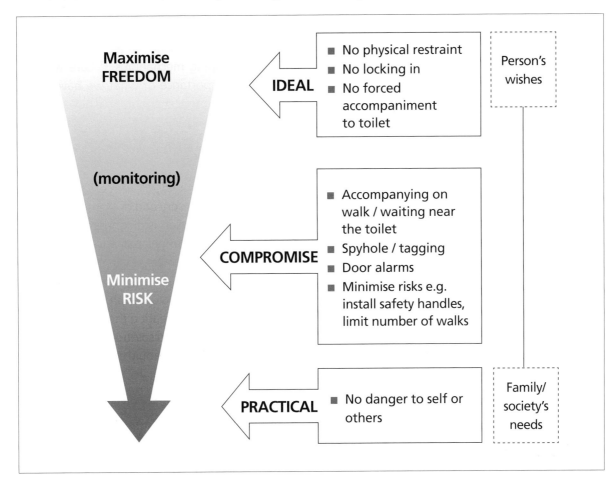

3.5   Moreover, the responses we received from our various consultative activities[120] suggest that the 'small' things – the 'micro' aspects of life and their effects – are of considerable significance both to autonomy and well-being. Quality of care and ethical issues are at least as much to do with the everyday as they are with the 'big' questions around the end of life. **How things are done, so that people with dementia feel valued individuals, will often be far more important than the particular structure or format of services.** These 'micro' aspects of care are often primarily a question of *attitude*, of professionals and care workers genuinely believing that the person with dementia for whom they are providing care matters as an individual, and is a 'person' in the fullest sense of the word. Such attitudes emerge in such mundane, everyday circumstances as whether a care worker in a residential setting checks whether the person with dementia would like sugar in their tea, or encourages them to express preferences in the clothes they put on in the morning.

3.6   The term *person-centred care* is widely used as a guiding principle in dementia care, following the pioneering work in dementia by Tom Kitwood, who argued both for the recognition of the 'person' in every individual, however advanced their dementia, and for the central place in dementia care of creating and sustaining meaningful relationships.[121] There were mixed, and to some extent polarised, views about the principle's value from respondents to our consultation, with some

---

[120] For example, in the Working Party's fact-finding visit to Vale House on 30 Sept 2008; see also Abbot W and Dugdale C (2005) It's the little things… *Journal of Dementia Care* **13(6)**: 12–4; Commission for Social Care Improvement (2008) *See Me, Not Just the Dementia: Understanding people's experiences of living in a care home* (London: CSCI).

[121] Kitwood T (1997) *Dementia Reconsidered: The person comes first* (Buckingham, UK: Open University Press).

concerns that over time the term had lost its original meaning and had become more associated with ideas of consumer choice. One respondent called it an idea that was initially "inspirational" but "now abused and ... exhausted by overuse."[122] Many found it bland or obvious. In so far as the term emphasises the importance of promoting each person's autonomy and well-being, it seems to us a useful concept. Any care which is genuinely tailored to the individual is likely to be culturally competent, in that it should take account of factors such as a person's language, religious beliefs and observance, cultural practices, social care support and coping mechanisms.[123] Care which is genuinely 'person-centred' may also help to emphasise the importance of what we have called the 'micro' aspects of life. We are aware, however, of the concern that the term may have become debased and used to describe almost any care, regardless of the extent to which it is based on a genuine relationship with, and concern for, the individual, and that therefore the term may have lost much of its original value as a guiding principle.

3.7 More recently, it has been argued that a *palliative care* approach would best support people with dementia. While for many, 'palliative' care is perceived as care at the very end of life, international definitions emphasise its applicability from the moment when a person is diagnosed with a life-threatening illness. The World Health Organization, for example, defines palliative care as "an approach that improves the quality of life of patients and their families facing the problems associated with life-threatening illness, through the prevention and relief of suffering by means of early identification and impeccable assessment and treatment of pain and other problems, physical, psychosocial and spiritual."[124] The emphasis placed in palliative care on treating the 'whole' person, not only their physical pain or difficulties, but also their mental, social and spiritual needs, is clearly relevant in the care of people with dementia, as is the emphasis that care should extend beyond the person with the illness to their family.

3.8 While the palliative care approach is widely admired, it is sometimes seen as relevant only when all attempts to 'cure' the person, or maintain their current state of health, have failed. In the context of cancer treatment, for example, a person may be referred for palliative care only when other forms of treatment are no longer possible or desirable. As a result, the idea of *supportive care* throughout an illness has been developed in order to avoid the stark distinction between 'active treatment' while a cure still seems possible and 'palliative care' when all hope of cure has been given up.[125] Instead, it is argued that supportive care, focusing on making the quality of the person's life as good as possible, should be provided throughout a person's illness, in addition to any available treatment for the disease itself. This concept of supportive care is clearly applicable to *any* serious condition which affects a person's quality of life; indeed, we were struck by how one person with dementia who gave evidence to the Working Party commented about the complete lack of supportive care she had received after her diagnosis, contrasting her situation with someone with a diagnosis of cancer.[126]

3.9 Those promoting supportive care suggest that, once a person has received a diagnosis of a life-threatening illness, the care and treatment provided should be thought of as consisting of three components:

[122] Professor June Andrews, Director, The Dementia Services Development Centre (DSDC), University of Stirling, responding to the Working Party's consultation.

[123] Iliffe S and Manthorpe J (2004) The debate on ethnicity and dementia: from category fallacy to person centred care? *Aging & Mental Health* **8(4)**: 283–92.

[124] For the World Health Organization's definition of palliative care, see: www.who.int/cancer/palliative/definition/en/.

[125] Ahmedzai SH (2005) The nature of palliation and its contribution to supportive care, in *Supportive Care in Respiratory Disease*, Ahmedzai SH and Muers MF (Editors) (Oxford: Oxford University Press), pp3–38; Ahmedzai SH and Walsh D (2000) Palliative medicine and modern cancer care *Seminars in Oncology* **27(1)**: 1–6; Hughes JC, Lloyd-Williams M and Sachs GA (Editors) (2010) *Supportive Care for the Person with Dementia* (Oxford: Oxford University Press, forthcoming).

[126] The Working Party's fact-finding meeting with people at the front-line of dementia care, 10 July 2008.

    1 *Disease-directed therapy*, which tackles the disorder itself;

    2. *Patient-directed care*, which covers the more general support the person might want or need, including pain relief, rehabilitation, practical and psychological support, and information;

    3. *Family-directed support*, which includes supporting the family in its caring role and also bereavement support after the patient's death.

'Supportive care' emphasises the importance of responding to the particular needs of the individual and those close to them, both in cases where treatment is available to tackle the underlying disorder and in cases where no such treatment as yet exists. It also emphasises the need to start support from the moment of diagnosis, again regardless of the availability of drug or other treatment to tackle the underlying disorder.

3.10 These three approaches – person-centred care, palliative care and supportive care – are all based on strong underpinning beliefs about the value of the person with dementia and the importance of all aspects of their being: their mental and physical well-being, their sense of self, their cultural and social background, their relationships, and their spiritual needs. The concept of supportive care appears to be particularly helpful in dementia, in that it emphasises the need to support both the person with dementia and their family, from the moment of diagnosis, regardless of the availability or appropriateness of treatment for the underlying brain disorder. In terms of our ethical framework, such supportive care recognises the value of the person with dementia and is concerned to promote the well-being and autonomy of that person while also paying attention to the interests of carers. However, we note that the 'label' attached to care is less important than the beliefs and attitudes underpinning that label. If care is provided on the basis that the person with dementia is valued as a person and supported to 'live well' with dementia, within the context of their own family and other relationships, then the label becomes immaterial.

3.11 A further issue stems from the importance of families and friends in the care of many people with dementia, as highlighted in the description of supportive care above. Most people with dementia are living in their own homes, with support from close relatives and friends. As we highlight in our discussion of solidarity (see paragraphs 2.43–2.47), an important aspect of the role of professionals is to provide support for *all* those affected, both in the sense of enabling the person with dementia to function and contribute as part of their family or social unit, and in the sense of providing support for family members and friends both in their caring role and in their own right. Indeed, in some older couples where one person has dementia and the other has other long-standing illnesses, there will be a strong element of interdependence: both may be 'carers' and 'cared-for' at the same time and need support for both aspects of their role.

3.12 During the consultation process we heard accounts from relatives where professionals appeared to treat them with suspicion or where information that would be useful in their caring role was not provided because of concerns about confidentiality.[127] We believe that an attitude of working *with* families and other carers, supporting them in their own care of the person with dementia, is more conducive to the interests of the person with dementia and better recognises the centrality of relationships with family and friends for many people with dementia. **We suggest that the appropriate attitude of professionals and care workers towards families should be that of *partners in care*, reflecting the solidarity being shown within the family**. Such a partnership would involve a relationship of trust between professionals and carers, based on mutual respect for each other's role and expertise. We return to this issue in more detail in Chapter 7 (see paragraphs 7.20–7.23).

---

127 Nuffield Council on Bioethics (2009) *Dementia: Ethical issues – summary of public consultation* (London: Nuffield Council on Bioethics), Q28.

3.13 High-quality support and care for people with dementia and their families can only become a reality if the interests of professionals and care workers are also properly considered. As we highlighted in Chapter 2 (see paragraph 2.42), those who provide formal care services need to be properly equipped to do their job through appropriate initial and ongoing education. There is, however, considerable evidence as to the lack of such dementia-specific education both in undergraduate professional training and for care workers who are expected to provide hands-on care for people with dementia.[128] The commitment to workforce development in both the English dementia strategy and Scottish dementia priority paper is therefore particularly welcome.[129] Moreover, working in dementia services will often be emotionally challenging, and a key part of the support people working in this field may need is access to some form of peer support network or 'caring community' where support and advice from those in similar situations may be sought.[130]

An ethical approach to a care pathway for people with dementia

Timing and communication of the diagnosis

"Early diagnosis is so important – so that I am involved in planning my future." *Nancy McAdam, consultation respondent*

"I was told very early that I have dementia. It was too early. My life would have been much easier without knowing my diagnosis." *Ernie Allan, consultation respondent*

"Admiral Nurses felt it was not so much about when the diagnosis was imparted (although we are clear it does need imparting as soon and as early as possible), it was more how it is imparted and how the person with dementia and their family are supported emotionally pre and post diagnosis." *Admiral Nurses – 'for dementia', consultation respondent*

Paul is 75. He is married to Marie, who is 73. For the last few months he has noticed that his memory is not what it used to be. He has had problems remembering names of people he knew well, and more recently with naming simple objects in the house. He has even forgotten a couple of bowls matches in which he was due to take part, and is becoming quite worried about his memory problems. He has mentioned these worries to Marie, but puts his problems down to the fact that he is just getting old. However, when his son came to stay last weekend with the grandchildren, his son said he should go and get a check-up with his GP. Paul is not too sure what to do. He tends to be quite pragmatic and get on with things and doesn't want to bother the doctor. However, if he is honest, he is also a bit scared. What if there is a problem and they cannot do anything about it? Wouldn't it be better to remain in ignorance? Or should he see someone in case something can be done to help him?

3.14 The prevailing view at present is that a diagnosis of dementia should be made as early as possible, and that it should be communicated directly to the individual, unless there are good reasons in a particular case to believe that the person would not want to know.[131] This approach was strongly supported by the majority, though not all, of the respondents to our consultation. We were told of many instances of the concerns of relatives or the person themselves that 'something was wrong' being incorrectly dismissed by general practitioners or hospital doctors. This left people

---

[128] See, for example, Dementia Services Development Centre, University of Stirling (2006) *The Need to Know: A survey of course input at pre-registration/undergraduate level on dementia* (Stirling: DSDC); All-Party Parliamentary Group on Dementia (2009) *Prepared to Care: Challenging the dementia skills gap* (London: Alzheimer's Society).

[129] Department of Health (2009) *Living Well with Dementia: A national dementia strategy* (London: Department of Health); NHS Scotland (2008) *Mental Health in Scotland: Dementia – A national priority summary paper* (Edinburgh: The Scottish Government).

[130] See, for example, Aase M, Nordrehaug and Malterud K (2008) "If you cannot tolerate that risk, you should never become a physician": a qualitative study about existential experiences among physicians *Journal of Medical* Ethics **34**: 767–71.

[131] See, for example, the English dementia strategy, summarised above and in Box 3.3; National Audit Office (2007) *Improving Services and Support for People with Dementia* (London: The Stationery Office), pp7–9; SIGN (2006) *Management of Patients with Dementia: A national clinical guideline* (Edinburgh: SIGN), paragraph 5.1.1.

with early dementia, and their families, without access to support. There are a number of benefits of early diagnosis, highlighted both by our respondents and in the research literature: the relief of understanding what is happening (both for the person with dementia and those close to him or her); the opportunity of accessing appropriate support services, including welfare benefits; the advantages of having time to plan; and the value of developing a trusting relationship with professionals.[132]

3.15 One problem at the very early stages of dementia is the uncertainty of diagnosis. It is currently very difficult to predict whether a person with 'mild cognitive impairment' will progress fairly rapidly to dementia, or whether they will never do so. Although there have been some developments in the use of biomarkers in this area,[133] it is not yet clear how results from small-scale studies in research centres will work in larger populations. Moreover, a reliable diagnosis may take some time, owing to the need to evaluate the implications and progress of the symptoms, and it may also be necessary to re-evaluate a provisional diagnosis in the light of new information. A wrong or premature diagnosis of dementia may lead simply to unnecessary distress and worry and indeed more practical difficulties, such as the potential loss of a person's driving licence or difficulties obtaining insurance.

3.16 Even where there is little doubt about the accuracy of the diagnosis, it cannot be assumed that *every* person with dementia will find that the advantages of early diagnosis and disclosure outweigh the disadvantages. A distinction between 'early' and 'timely' diagnosis is helpful in this respect.[134] As the Alzheimer's Society noted in its response to our consultation: "for conveying a diagnosis to be helpful and appropriate, it must be timely, with benefits balanced against risks. Where a person stands to be distressed to the point where no benefit can be derived, then even an early diagnosis is perhaps not a timely one." This approach is in line with our own emphasis on considering both the well-being and the autonomy of the person with dementia: where the person is not seeking a diagnosis, and where their well-being is unlikely to be enhanced by the diagnosis, then it is inappropriate to force that diagnosis upon them.

3.17 However, while recognising this distinction between 'early' and 'timely' diagnosis, it is crucial not to make assumptions about the effect the diagnosis will have on the person with dementia. Recent research has suggested that the vast majority of people with mild dementia *do* wish to be informed about their diagnosis (even if family members think they do not), and that fears as to the impact of this information on the person's general mental health are generally unfounded.[135] It seems likely that a 'timely' diagnosis for most people will be the point when the cognitive and other changes they are experiencing begin to have a significant effect on their lives or on the lives of those close to them.

3.18 **We conclude that people should have access to good quality assessment and support from the time they, or their families, become concerned about symptoms that relate to a possible diagnosis of dementia.** We welcome the fact that improvements in early intervention and diagnosis are highlighted in the Scottish dementia priority paper[136] and included as one of the seven "key priority

[132] Nuffield Council on Bioethics (2009) *Dementia: Ethical issues – summary of public consultation* (London: Nuffield Council on Bioethics), Q6; Bamford C, Lamont S, Eccles M et al. (2004) Disclosing a diagnosis of dementia: a systematic review *International Journal of Geriatric Psychiatry* **19(2)**: 151–69.

[133] Hansson O, Zetterberg H, Buchhave P et al. (2006) Association between CSF biomarkers and incipient Alzheimer's disease in patients with mild cognitive impairment: a follow up study *Lancet Neurology* **5(3)**: 228–34.

[134] Alzheimer's Society, responding to the Working Party's consultation.

[135] See, for example, Carpenter BD, Xiong C, Porensky EK et al. (2008) Reaction to a dementia diagnosis in individuals with Alzheimer's disease and mild cognitive impairment *Journal of the American Geriatrics Society* **56**: 405–12; Pinner G and Boulman WP (2003) Attitudes of patients with mild dementia and their carers towards disclosure of the diagnosis *International Psychogeriatrics* **15(3)**: 279–88.

[136] NHS Scotland (2008) *Mental Health in Scotland: Dementia – A national priority summary paper* (Edinburgh: The Scottish Government).

outcomes" in the English dementia strategy.[137] We caution, however, that the timeliness of a diagnosis will depend on the person and family concerned. We also emphasise that uncertainties about diagnosis should never be used as an excuse not to communicate openly with a person who is aware of changes in themselves and is actively seeking explanations. Respect for that person's well-being and autonomy demands an honest response. As we note in Chapter 1 (see paragraph 1.36), there is no value at present in attempting to screen for the underlying disease processes in the brain before symptoms of dementia appear.

3.19 There is some evidence to suggest that people in some cultural groups may be more hesitant in coming forward for diagnosis than those from other cultural groups.[138] Although individual choices and differences should be respected, it is important, given the benefits of earlier diagnosis noted in paragraph 3.14, to understand the reasons that prevent people from coming forward. We suspect that feelings of shame and stigma associated with dementia (see Chapter 4) play an important part in these reasons and that their significance varies between cultures. There are also concerns as to potential cultural bias in some of the cognitive tests used in the process of diagnosing dementia.[139]

Recommendation 1: We recommend that the UK Departments of Health should encourage more research to be carried out on the reasons why there is variation between cultures in readiness to come forward for diagnosis, and the role that misinformation and misunderstanding plays in these reasons.

3.20 The *way* in which a diagnosis is conveyed is clearly also important and is a key aspect of demonstrating respect for the personhood and well-being of the person with dementia. Research published in 2008 highlighted the lack of sensitivity with which a diagnosis is sometimes conveyed, with participants in the research describing how they were treated in an uncaring and unsympathetic manner: being told "well it's Alzheimer's, what do you expect?"; or being given the diagnosis over the phone by someone they had never previously met.[140] It is also important that the disclosure of a diagnosis of dementia is not just seen as a one-off event, but rather as a *process*, starting with the point when the person is first referred for assessment and continuing on into follow-up support once the diagnosis itself has been established.[141] We consider this issue of follow-up further below (see paragraphs 3.25–3.29).

3.21 Finally there is the question of to whom the diagnosis should be given: should close family members or other carers also be informed? Responses to our consultation included several examples where doctors assessed the person with suspected dementia but, on grounds of confidentiality, gave little or no information to relatives.[142]

3.22 Whilst the principle of patient confidentiality is an important one in the doctor–patient relationship, a diagnosis of dementia has implications not only for the person with dementia, but also for close family members who are likely to take on a significant caring role and need appropriate information and support to do so. Moreover, the assessment of possible early dementia requires information

---

[137] Department of Health (2009) *Living Well with Dementia: The national dementia strategy implementation plan* (London: Department of Health), paragraph 2.1.

[138] See, for example, La Fontaine J, Ahuja J, Bradbury NM, Phillips S and Oyebode JR (2007) Understanding dementia amongst people in minority ethnic and cultural groups *Journal of Advanced Nursing* **60(6)**: 605–14.

[139] Rait G and Burns A (1998) Screening for depression and cognitive impairment in older people from ethnic minorities *Age and Ageing* **27**: 271–5; Shah A (1999) Difficulties experienced by a Gujarati geriatric psychiatrist in interviewing Gujarati elders in Gujarati *International Journal of Geriatric Psychiatry* **14**: 1072–4; Bowes A and Wilkinson H (2003) 'We didn't know it would get that bad': South Asian experiences of dementia and the service response *Health and Social Care in the Community* **11**: 387–96.

[140] Alzheimer's Society (2008) *Dementia: Out of the shadows* (London: Alzheimer's Society), p22.

[141] Fisk JD, Beattie BL, Donnelly M, Byszewski A and Molnar FJ (2007) Disclosure of the diagnosis of dementia *Alzheimer's & Dementia* **3**: 404–10.

[142] For example Agnes Charnley, responding to the Working Party's consultation.

from those close to the person with possible dementia, both about their own awareness of changes in the person's behaviour and cognitive performance, and about any difficulties which family and friends are themselves experiencing. A person even in the early stages of dementia may not give an accurate account of what difficulties they or their family members face, and what care needs are present. This may be compounded by poor insight into the problems.

3.23 **We conclude that professionals responsible for communicating a diagnosis of dementia should actively encourage the person with dementia to share this information with their family, making clear that the diagnosis is of importance to those providing informal care and support, as well as to the individual concerned.** Practical ways in which professionals could promote information sharing in this way include encouraging the person to attend appointments with a friend or family member they trust, so that all information is given to both parties together; being willing to listen to those concerned about the person with dementia; and if necessary acting as an intermediary within the family.

3.24 If the person with dementia refuses absolutely to allow information to be shared with others, this refusal must be honoured while the person has the capacity to make this decision. However, the professionals involved should make clear to the person with dementia that it may be necessary to share information with others later, once capacity to make this decision has been lost, in the interests of the person's own well-being (see further discussion of this issue at paragraphs 7.24–7.26). Professionals should also in such cases consider the issue of capacity very carefully, as inability to "understand the information relevant to the decision" (for example by being in denial over the diagnosis) may, under the Mental Capacity Act, mean that the person does not have legal capacity to make this decision. Nevertheless, it should be emphasised that both the Mental Capacity Act and the Adults with Incapacity (Scotland) Act protect a person's right to make unwise or risky decisions, as long as they retain the capacity to do so.

Recommendation 2: We recommend that the General Medical Council and relevant royal colleges, including the Royal College of Psychiatrists, the Royal College of Physicians, the Royal College of General Practitioners and the Royal College of Nursing, should consider ways of promoting an approach to the disclosure of a diagnosis of dementia that acknowledges the role of those close to the person with dementia, for example through the production of guidance on family involvement and confidentiality at the point of diagnosis.

Information, communication and signposting to services

"[The support needed most is] adequate provision of information … relating to both the disease process itself, the diagnosis, the likely progression and prognosis, the treatment options and availability and access to care networks." *British Geriatrics Society, consultation respondent*

"The support needed most is more advice strategies to deal with confusion and anxiety. I appreciate that everyone behaves differently but I do believe that there are common traits and it seems to be that every carer is learning the hard way from personal experience." *Mrs Linda Tolson, consultation respondent*

Paul has been given a diagnosis of early dementia. He went to his GP, who asked him some questions and then sent him along to the local memory clinic. Here he saw a nurse and a doctor and had a few other tests done, including a brain scan. His wife, Marie, was there when he was given the diagnosis, which was helpful because he forgot quickly what the doctor said. The question now is what can be done? What support is available to him and also to Marie? What is likely to happen to him? How bad will the dementia get and how quickly? Who can help them navigate the implications of this difficult diagnosis? And what should he tell his children?

3.25 The importance of information, support and access to services immediately after diagnosis has been emphasised in a number of recent reports and guidelines, and was evident in the responses we received to our public consultation.[143] Information that people find helpful includes factual information about particular forms of dementia, advice and counselling from professionals, tips on practical strategies for dealing with difficult situations or behaviours, and details about the availability both of peer support networks and other local statutory and voluntary services. Clearly, the information needs of any one person with dementia and those close to them will vary significantly, depending both on personal preference and on the nature and progress of their dementia at the point of diagnosis. A physically active person with early-onset dementia who is still in employment at the time of diagnosis is likely to have very different information and support needs compared with a much older person who already has some degree of community support from the NHS or social services because of existing physical health needs or general frailty.

3.26 There is, however, ample evidence that, in many cases, people are presented with a diagnosis of dementia and simply told to come back in a year's time.[144] **It was argued forcefully in one of our fact-finding meetings with people in front-line dementia care that such a lack of information and support in the immediate aftermath of diagnosis is simply morally wrong.**[145] We agree. We argue in Chapter 2 that people with dementia are of equal value to people without dementia, that their autonomy and well-being interests are important, and that some support may well be necessary in order to promote and protect those interests. It is clear from the reports cited above, the Department of Health's consultation on the English dementia strategy, and the responses to our own consultation, that access to supportive care, including appropriate information, emotional support, and a variety of forms of practical support, is essential for people to live well with dementia, making the most of all their retained abilities.

3.27 People also need help in accessing what is inevitably a fragmented support system, given the wide range of health and social services which people with dementia and their families may potentially use. Such support may take many forms, but we suggest that a key element will be the identification of a single individual to liaise with the person with dementia and their family, and with whom a trusting relationship can develop. **We welcome the proposal in the English dementia strategy to pilot possible models of 'dementia care advisers', whose role would be to help people diagnosed with dementia access appropriate services and support. We suggest that there is a strong ethical justification for such a role to be introduced throughout the UK as soon as possible.**

3.28 Moreover, the importance of *communication* itself should not be underestimated. A common fear about dementia is the fear of being cut off from others, no longer able to communicate and relate to them in the way we have done in the past. An equally common misconception about dementia is the idea that, because spoken conversation becomes more difficult as the dementia progresses, communication itself becomes impossible. On the contrary, we believe that communication is indeed possible and that a key aspect of recognising and relating to the person with dementia is to find appropriate forms of communication through which they may be reached, however advanced their dementia may have become. Moreover, it has been argued that the extent to which decisions about people with dementia are likely to be right or good may depend on the extent to which communication between all concerned (the person with dementia, professionals, family and friends) is open, free and based on mutual respect.[146]

---

[143] NICE/SCIE (2006) *Dementia: Supporting people with dementia and their carers in health and social care*, NICE Clinical Guideline 42 (London: NICE and SCIE); NHS Scotland (2008) *Mental health in Scotland: Dementia – A national priority summary paper* (Edinburgh: The Scottish Government); Nuffield Council on Bioethics (2009) *Dementia: Ethical issues – summary of public consultation* (London: Nuffield Council on Bioethics), Q1.

[144] See, for example, National Audit Office (2007) *Improving Services and Support for People with Dementia* (London: The Stationery Office), pp30–1; Alzheimer's Society (2008) *Dementia: Out of the shadows* (London: Alzheimer's Society), pp22–5.

[145] The Working Party's fact-finding meeting with people at the front-line of dementia care, 10 July 2008.

[146] Moody HR (1992) *Ethics in an Aging Society* (Baltimore: Johns Hopkins University Press).

3.29 The examples of practice outlined in Boxes 3.5–3.9 below illustrate what can be done in terms of information, advice and communication, to help people come to terms with their diagnosis, access the help and support they need, and continue to feel part of a social community.

Box 3.5: Example from practice – diagnosis and subsequent information and support

Newbury Memory Clinic, which is run in a GP surgery by the mental health trust old age psychiatry unit, offers holistic diagnosis and advice in the community. A diagnosis of dementia at the clinic is immediately followed by a meeting with the memory clinic nurse, who counsels the person with dementia and their carer and provides them with written information. They then meet with an adviser/counsellor from the clinic to inform them of a range of support networks and therapeutic activities.

Cited in: National Audit Office (2007) *Improving Services and Support for People with Dementia* (London: The Stationery Office), p29.

Box 3.6: Example from practice – post-diagnostic support system in the Stewartry area of Dumfries and Galloway

A partnership between **Alzheimer Scotland** and the **community mental health team (CMHT) in Dumfries and Galloway** provides early-stage support to people with a diagnosis of dementia, both through the provision of memory groups, and through personal support for people with dementia and their carers by a member of the CMHT. A key part of the programme is the use of a checklist, used at the person's own speed, which covers issues such as assessment, diagnosis, further information and explanation, medication, social impact, current support, carer assessment, challenging behaviour, relationship issues and welfare. Once all these issues have been 'ticked off' the list, the person with dementia and their carers should have a clear idea of where they can get help, if they need or want it. After this, there is continued support from the CMHT, from external agencies such as Alzheimer Scotland, and from social services, including access to a carer education and support course specifically aimed at carers 12–18 months after diagnosis.

More information from: Alzheimer Scotland, Dumfries and Galloway services, www.alzscot.org/pages/regions/dumfries.htm; **telephone 01387 261303.**

Box 3.7: Example from practice – psychological support and education for people with dementia and their families

Alzheimer Cafés provide a monthly gathering where persons with dementia and/or their family and friends can be together in a safe, welcoming environment, in the company of other carers, local Alzheimer support group members, volunteers, and health and social care professionals, for the purpose of emotional support, education and social interaction.

A typical evening at the Café starts with music and socialising over light refreshments. A presentation or interview about a theme linked with dementia then follows by a professional or family member with hands-on experience of the subject being discussed. The evening continues with further social interaction, refreshments and the opportunity to speak informally with the guest speaker or professionals present. Twice a year, purely social evenings are held with live music or other entertainment.

More information from: www.alzheimercafe.co.uk/What.htm.

Box 3.8: Example from practice – reaching people who might not otherwise access services

Bradford-based project **'Meri Yaadain'** raises awareness of dementia among Bradford's South Asian communities and encourages people with dementia and carers to access information, support and services. It includes a monthly support group with culturally appropriate activities and currently supports over 80 families, including providing advocacy support to ensure that local health and social services meet people's cultural and language needs.

More information from: www.alzheimers.org.uk/downloads/LWD_sep_08_low_res.pdf.

Box 3.9: Example from practice – good communication as speech becomes more difficult

Researchers at the **Augmentative and Alternative Communication (AAC) unit** at the University of Stirling have developed Talking Mats™, a low-technology communication framework for with people with dementia.

Talking Mats™ uses a textured mat and a system of simple picture symbols that are placed on the mat as conversation with a person with dementia progresses. Each picture offers the person with dementia the opportunity to express their feelings about four aspects of their well-being (activities; people; environment; and self) by placing the relevant image below a visual scale based on levels of happiness.[147]

More information from: www.talkingmats.com/.

---

[147] Murphy J, Gray CM and Cox S (2007) *Communication and Dementia: How Talking Mats can help people with dementia to express themselves* (York: Joseph Rowntree Foundation), pp6–7; AAC Research Unit, University of Stirling, responding to the Working Party's consultation.

Ongoing care and support

"Practical assistance is only one part of the support required by a person with dementia. There is also a need for emotional happiness, stimulation and social interaction." *Alzheimer's Society, consultation respondent*

"Support must focus on enabling the person, and those around them, to sustain skills and to draw upon the strengths within their personality and previous experience." *British Geriatrics Society, consultation respondent*

"Visiting a home for elderly people during my mental health block, I found that the home was more suited for people with a British background, from the décor, to the ballads from the 60s and 70s ... Would someone from a different culture really be able to enjoy themselves here?" *Member of the special study group on dementia, Leicester University, consultation respondent*

Roy is a 67-year-old man with mild multi-infarct dementia. He has been up and down quite a bit over the last few months, but generally copes well with the support of his partner, Doreen. He does tend to forget things, and every now and then can be a bit confused. Doreen and Roy have been together 20 years. Roy's family have very little to do with him, but Doreen's son and partner are very supportive of them both, popping round once or twice a week. The support is more emotional than practical, although they do take Roy and Doreen away with them on holiday every year. Derek, who is a member of a local voluntary care in the community organisation, goes out with Roy once or twice a week. They often go to the local football match, and, if the weather is good, fishing. This gives Doreen the time she needs to get the shopping and have her hair done, and Roy is able to continue with his lifelong interests. Derek will come round to stay with Roy when Doreen has to go out at other times, for example when she goes to her hospital appointment. Roy has got to know Derek well, and enjoys his company.

Winston is an 83-year-old man of West Indian origin. He was diagnosed with dementia four years ago, and the disorder has progressed quite rapidly. He needs a lot of help with self care, and with feeding. He needs escorting to the toilet. He currently lives with his 58-year-old daughter, Vanessa, and her partner. He attends a day centre two days a week. He also spends two weeks in residential care every three months, to give Vanessa time for a break, and give him a rest too. Vanessa has just picked her father up from a two-week stay in the care home, and been told that he seems to be off his food. He has been seen by the doctor, and there does not appear to be any physical cause for this. When Vanessa gets him home, he seems to regain his usual very good appetite. She wonders what has been going on. Is he unhappy in the home? Is it because the staff at the home seem to have changed again? Or does he just like her cooking? She does tend to make him some of his favourite West Indian dishes. Or might it be that he enjoys meal times where she spends a long time with him helping him to eat his food in a quiet environment?

3.30 We have stressed the importance, if care is to be of appropriately high ethical standards, of support that promotes the autonomy and well-being of the person with dementia and that recognises their individuality and value as a person. NICE has made a number of recommendations in these areas, emphasising the importance of promoting independence and helping maintain a person's skills, responding flexibly to fluctuating abilities, providing care in a stable and familiar environment, and enabling the person to participate in activities which they enjoy. The English dementia strategy similarly stresses the importance of community personal support services "ranging from early intervention to specialist home care services, which are responsive to the personal needs and preferences of each individual and take account of broader family circumstances."[148] The strategy further highlights the role of housing and housing support services in supporting people with dementia to live in their own homes for as long as possible, and the importance of ensuring people are able to 'live well' with dementia in care homes.[149]

3.31 **We very much welcome the increasing emphasis on services which are flexible and appropriate to the individual and which enable them to live well with dementia – an approach based on respect for the needs, preferences and personhood of the individual person with dementia.**

[148] Department of Health (2009) *Living Well with Dementia: A national dementia strategy* (London: Department of Health), p46.
[149] *Ibid*, pp55–61.

Clearly, the development of a particular level of high-quality services will be dependent in part on resources, both in terms of money and in terms of a workforce with the appropriate skills and, as we discuss in Chapter 4 (see paragraph 4.38), we hesitate to make specific recommendations with economic implications which we are not well placed to consider. However, a commitment to making services as flexible and responsive as possible does not necessarily entail spending more money; rather, it involves listening to the needs and wishes of the person for whom the service is being provided and adjusting the support on offer in order to help them in what *they* value most. Some people who have difficulty doing their own shopping, for example, may prefer to go shopping with a home care worker, rather than having the shopping done for them.[150] Similarly, in some cases where the person with dementia needs more intimate personal care in the home, in terms of washing, dressing and using the toilet, but has a carer able and willing to provide this support, the person and their family may best be supported by offering other forms of assistance instead of insisting that only personal care is available. Responding to need with this degree of flexibility does not necessarily involve increasing budgets, or making difficult trade-offs between the needs of one group and the needs of another.

> **Box 3.10: Example from practice – 'In control' approach in East Renfrewshire**
>
> **Alzheimer Scotland** is launching a new post-diagnosis project in East Renfrewshire and Renfrewshire. Supported by the Scottish Government, the project will help people with early dementia to come to terms with their diagnosis, and will support them to find their own ways of maintaining their network and natural supports instead of being offered a single package of 'care'. The project will also support people to use 'advanced person-centred planning' to design future support using individual budgets over which they have personal control.
>
> **More information:** www.alzscot.org/downloads/dis65.pdf.

3.32 We also highlight the high value to be placed upon developing relationships with individual care workers, particularly those working in the person's own home. In one of our fact-finding meetings, for example, we heard of one person with dementia who received home care from 14 different people over a period of eight months.[151] While some degree of staff turnover is inevitable, examples such as these suggest that the importance to the person with dementia of personal relationships, particularly where intimate care is being provided, has been given little consideration or priority in the planning of some services. Indeed, there is some evidence to suggest that support for home care workers – such as regular meetings with other team members where information can be shared and discussed – and access to training, may make it easier for services to retain their staff.[152] Such support for staff not only acknowledges the importance of the interests of staff being given weight for their own sake (see paragraph 2.42), but is also likely to have a positive effect on the autonomy and well-being of the person with dementia.

3.33 As we discuss above (see paragraph 3.5), the 'small things' of care are extremely important in ensuring that care is genuinely supportive of the individual, and enhances a person's autonomy and well-being. The humanity with which assistance for everyday living is offered, especially help with eating and intimate care, is crucial in helping the person retain their self-esteem and dignity, as are the manner and tone in which a person is addressed; the care taken to ensure that they participate as much as they can or wish in any decision about their day-to-day life; the trouble taken about appropriate and attractive food and environments; and access to meaningful activity. We note in Box 3.13 below some examples of how these 'small things' may be achieved in practice.

---

[150] Snayde F and Moriarty J (2009) Person-centred home-care for people with dementia: developing a specialist service in an ethnically diverse community *Dementia* **8(1):** 148–52.

[151] The Working Party's fact-finding meeting with people at the front-line of dementia care, 10 July 2008.

[152] Snayde F and Moriarty J (2009) Person-centred home-care for people with dementia: developing a specialist service in an ethnically diverse community *Dementia* **8(1):** 148–52. See also Vernooij-Dassen MJ, Faber MJ and Olde Rikkert MG (2009) Dementia care and labour market: the role of job satisfaction *Aging & Mental Health* **13(3):** 383–90.

3.34 In Chapter 2 we suggested that the idea of treating a person with dignity can be helpful in the setting of dementia care and this is perhaps particularly true with regard to helping people with their personal and physical care needs. When people complain that a person with dementia has been treated in an undignified manner, it is often with respect to some aspect of physical care such as toileting or dressing; or the way in which a person is spoken to authoritatively or patronisingly, or alternatively left alone and ignored. The concept of dignity is useful, we believe, in highlighting both the autonomy and well-being of the person with dementia. If a person with dementia is neither able to express how they would like to be treated, nor to complain about how they are being treated, then it may be difficult to judge what should be done. The concept of dignity can be helpful in highlighting that it remains important, even in very severe dementia, to think carefully about the interests and feelings of the person. Treating a person with dignity involves a compassionate understanding of what the person is likely to be experiencing, and respecting the views and values that they previously held.

3.35 The notion of treating a person with dignity can thus be helpful in ensuring that a person is not ignored or left in an inappropriate state. But thought still needs to be given to what is meant by 'dignity' in a particular situation, and this involves, in our view, careful consideration of both a person's autonomy and their well-being. For example, a person with dementia in a care home who tends to remain in their own bedroom may in some cases be actively choosing privacy, but in others they may remain there simply because they cannot remember where they are, or how to find the lounge without becoming lost and distressed. Similar difficulties may arise in helping a person with their choice of clothes: is the goal to make the person look normal or dress in their characteristic way, or to help them be comfortable, or to let them choose for themselves even at the risk that their choices may make them conspicuous or provoke criticism? Although there is no straightforward answer to these questions, the idea of dignity alone seems insufficient. Some balancing of various interests – the person's previous views, current wishes, and well-being interests – is needed in this situation.

> ### Box 3.11: Example from practice – support in everyday activities
>
> "I was put in touch with Neil, a befriender. We meet twice a week. We have a good understanding and trust one another. Our meetings are good fun. Neil doesn't tell me where to go – I ask and he takes me. He'd never been fishing but he took it up to please me. I'd never been bowling, so he took me."
>
> JDI Mutual Support Group (2008) *In the Mists of Memory — A celebration of the circle of life* (Falkirk: Joint Dementia Initiative), p47.

> ### Box 3.12: Example from practice – support in the community
>
> **Guideposts Trust** Specialist Dementia Home Care Service has been developed with Warwickshire Social Services to provide a specialist, needs-led and person-centred dementia domiciliary service. It:
>
> - provides support within people's own homes;
> - enables people with dementia to maximise their lives through identifying their strengths and abilities; and
> - facilitates hospital discharge, helping people remain in their own homes and reducing unnecessary admission to 24-hour residential care.
>
> Guideposts Dementia Home Care Service, telephone: **01788 577825. See:** www.guidepoststrust.org.uk/warwickshire/index.php?page=specialist_dementia.
>
> **Dementia Care Partnership** (DCP) is a charity based in Newcastle-upon-Tyne. Formerly the Dementia Care Initiative, it provides local services for people with dementia and their carers. DCP aims to offer community-based alternatives to residential care. It offers people with dementia and their carers services such as home support, day activity centres, supported-living houses in partnership with social and housing services, a 24-hour companion and befriender scheme, and residential short term breaks.
>
> DCP has also established The Bradbury Centre, a facility for people with dementia and their carers (and also open to the general public) that incorporates services such as a café, a hairdresser, a health and fitness room, a multi-faith room, and a training and conference facility.
>
> Dementia Care Partnership: www.dementiacare.org.uk/html/about_us.html. **See also** Garwood S (2009) Partnership in word and deed *Journal of Dementia Care* **17(1)**: 20–4.

Box 3.13: Example from practice – residential care

Vale House in Oxford is a purpose-built specialist care home, caring for 20 people with dementia. The admission criteria are that the person has dementia, is (usually) over 60 years old, and has behavioural difficulties (such as very loud or aggressive behaviour) which cannot be managed elsewhere. The philosophy of the home (described by the Head of Home as 'the reason why we're doing this') includes:

■ respecting the 'adult status' of the person with dementia;

■ helping people with dementia live their lives as independently as possible, making full use of their remaining capacities;

■ recognising that feelings matter every moment of the day;

■ focusing on providing comfort and support; and

■ acting in a 'person-centred way' to colleagues as well as residents.

Important aspects of living up to this philosophy include finding out as much as possible about the person with dementia before they move into the home, training staff to be very aware of the importance of 'little things' like smiling and talking softly, and liaising closely with families.

Vale House, Oxford: www.valehouse.org.uk.

Box 3.14: Example from practice – dementia-specific design in residential care

A range of visuoperceptual and orientation difficulties often occur in dementia, in addition to normal visual difficulties associated with age. Ideas such as those below are increasingly being promoted:

For care:

■ Help with activities and socialisation: for example adapting the layout of communal rooms into smaller, social groupings, so that people can see and hear each other better; providing a variety of types of seating to suit a person's choice of activity; and providing alternatives to constant television, such as an aquarium or calming DVD images.

■ Ensuring that residents are not startled when staff approach them – for example by approaching from the front, or speaking first.

■ Use of strong colours for crockery and cups: in one study, a group of people with advanced Alzheimer's disease ate nearly 25 per cent more than usual when offered meals on bright red crockery and drank over 80 per cent more than usual when offered drinks in bright red cups, compared with the original white.[153]

For more appropriate environments:

■ Appropriate use of bright and strongly contrasting colours to highlight important features such as toilet doors, toilet seats, handrails and steps.

■ Provision of good levels of lighting to eliminate shadows and promote mobility.

■ Use of colour and design to encourage orientation, for example using different colours, or particular types of artwork, to identify different parts of the building.

■ Avoiding use of reflective surfaces and mirrors which may easily be misinterpreted, and strongly patterned surfaces.

For more information on design recommendation, see Jones GMM and van der Eerden WJ (2008) Designing care environments for persons with Alzheimer's disease: visuoperceptual considerations *Reviews in Clinical Gerontology* **18**: 13–37. The Dementia Services Development at Stirling University has developed a gold standard award scheme for dementia-friendly design, with the first award made in 2008 to The Lodge (dementia care facility) at Buckshaw Retirement Village.

Box 3.15: Example from practice – services for people with learning disabilities and dementia

Bourne Cottage in Ewell, Surrey, is a specialist day service run by Surrey Council's adult social care department for people with dementia and learning disabilities. The cottage is open on a daily basis to people with learning disabilities and dementia who have become distressed when attending their usual, busier day services.

The cottage hosts around ten people with learning disabilities and dementia each day, offering facilities such as a sensory garden and opportunities to participate in reminiscence activities in a comfortable, manageable environment. Although the cottage welcomes carers of those who visit the cottage, they are not obliged to accompany the person for whom they care.

More information: Dr Karen Dodd, Surrey and Borders Partnership NHS Foundation Trust (drkaren.dodd@sabp.nhs.uk).

Box 3:16: Example from practice – enhancing lives

Music for Life is a partnership between the organisation **'for dementia'** and **Wigmore Hall**. The project works with people with dementia and the staff who care for them in a variety of settings. Professional musicians use improvisation to draw out the potential of people with dementia for self-expression and communication, particularly helping those who are emotionally isolated and disempowered as a result of the advanced stage of their condition.

More information: www.wigmore-hall.org.uk/community-and-education/musicforlife and www.fordementia.org.uk/.

---

[153] Dunne T, Neargarder S, Cipolloni P and Cronin-Golomb A (2004) Visual contrast enhances food and liquid intake in advanced Alzheimer's disease *Clinical Nutrition* **23(4)**: 533–8.

Acute hospital services

"My mother became bed-bound for a few weeks on going into hospital. Physiotherapy was arranged to help to get her mobile again. She was denied help because no one could give her any physical support, so no one could help her out of her chair, and also because she was in some pain, and said 'no'. She never walked again." *Anonymous consultation respondent*

"… A patient with dementia who is admitted to an acute ward following an infection or fall finds themselves being repeatedly transferred from one ward to another, and from one bed to another … The hospital then express surprise or outrage when the patient who has been moved around like a parcel becomes frightened and protests loudly, or gets into the wrong bed by mistake." *Anonymous consultation respondent*

> Farah is 78 years old. She has Alzheimer's disease, and is currently living in a residential home. She copes very well but does have a tendency to 'wander'. Her daughter, Priya, lives nearby and visits two or three times a week. The rest of the family live further away. Farah has a possible skin cancer on her arm that needs to be removed. However, she is likely to get confused by the trip to the hospital. Priya is concerned as her last trip with her mother to the hospital, following a fall in which she fractured her wrist, was not a good one. Her mother became very agitated during the three-hour wait to be seen in casualty and the staff did not know how to deal with her behaviour.

3.36 People with dementia often require medical assessment, services and treatment that are not directly related to their dementia: for example, they may need to attend an accident and emergency department after a fall, or be admitted into hospital for an orthopaedic operation or for treatment of a serious infection. Respondents to our consultation gave examples of difficulties that people with dementia and carers sometimes experience through lack of knowledge on the part of some health professionals about dementia, and also through lack of arrangements in hospitals for enabling people with dementia to be properly assessed and treated for these independent medical conditions. For example, hospital staff sometimes interpreted behaviour linked with the dementia, such as wandering off, as evidence that the person was refusing or avoiding assessment, with the result that proper assessments were not carried out; or hospitals were inflexible in not understanding or allowing for the problems of fear and confusion that can be particularly problematic for people with dementia, for example by not allowing relatives to stay with the person with dementia.[154]

3.37 Not only do such experiences cause significant (and often avoidable) distress at the time to people with dementia and their carers: there is also evidence to suggest that the disorientation and distress that people with dementia often experience in hospital have a long-term and permanent effect on the person's cognitive abilities and capacity to continue coping on their own.[155] Indeed, a hospital admission will often be a 'trigger' for admission into residential care, thus forcing the person with dementia and those close to them to make important decisions about the future at a point of crisis, instead of in their own time.[156]

3.38 Although there were accounts of problems, we also came across areas of good practice and we describe some of these in Boxes 3.17 and 3.18 below. As we note at the beginning of this Chapter (see paragraph 3.1), there may be good reasons why an innovative solution that works well in one area may not simply transfer elsewhere, and more research comparing different models for supporting people with dementia appropriately in hospital is needed (see Recommendation 16

---

[154] Nuffield Council on Bioethics (2009) *Dementia: Ethical issues – summary of public consultation* (London: Nuffield Council on Bioethics), Q21.

[155] Borbasi S, Jones J, Lockwood C and Emden C (2006) Health professionals' perspectives of providing care to people with dementia in the acute setting: toward better practice *Geriatric Nursing* **27(5)**: 300–8.

[156] See, for example, Ballard C, Clack H and Green D (2007) Postoperative cognitive decline, dementia and anaesthesia *British Journal of Hospital Medicine* **68(11)**: 576–7; Holmes J and House A (2000) Psychiatric illness predicts poor outcome after surgery for hip fracture: a prospective cohort study *Psychological Medicine* **30**: 921–9.

after paragraph 8.18). The English dementia strategy promotes the idea of specialist liaison older people's mental health teams in general hospitals, but notes that there is considerable diversity in the models currently adopted and highlights the need for a thorough review of the evidence base.[157] It seems to us that, whatever model of support is chosen, there will be at least two features which will be essential to its success: first, staff who are knowledgeable about dementia; and, secondly, an underpinning belief that people with dementia are fully 'persons' who are entitled to the same level of good medical care as anyone else.

> **Box 3.17: Example from practice – providing support in A&E**
>
> The Accident and Emergency Department at **Southampton University Hospitals NHS Trust** includes a team providing specialist assistance to people with dementia. The team aims to identify people with dementia (with or without a diagnosis) who attend A&E for reasons such as a fall. They are able to offer a quiet space within the A&E department to take histories from both the person with dementia and their carer, allowing as much time as is necessary. They are then able to make direct contact with relevant services such as community services, GPs, equipment stores and Community Mental Health Teams, in order to avoid inappropriate admissions, while recognising that in some cases admissions will be appropriate.
>
> **More information:** Nadia.Chambers@suht.swest.nhs.uk.

> **Box 3.18: Example from practice – specialist GP support to care homes**
>
> **Dr Gillie Evans** works as a GP at the **Jenner Health Centre** in Whittlesey, Cambridgeshire. She provides dedicated GP services to 50 residents with moderate and severe dementia living in a care home in her local area.
>
> Since 2002, Dr Evans has taken a personal list approach to the care of these residents, visiting on a weekly basis for a full morning session. She is supported in this approach by the home manager and all the staff. A member of the nursing staff accompanies her and communicates with relatives after her visit.
>
> **More information from:** www.dementia.jennerhealthcentre.co.uk/.

End of life palliative care

"… we know people with dementia can be deprived of even basic palliative care."
Admiral Nurses – 'for dementia', consultation respondent

> John has severe dementia. In his working life he managed a large department in a production factory, doing a great deal of national and international travel. Control and personal autonomy were very important to him. In conversations about the end of life with his family he said that if he were to become a 'cabbage' the family were to 'switch the machine off'. Yet, once he began to be affected by dementia, he found things to enjoy, particularly his family and grandchildren. Now, although confined to bed and having to be turned regularly to prevent bed sores, he still remains at home cared for by his wife, district nurses and care workers. His life is in its end stages. He appears to be comfortable and not in pain, and seems to enjoy familiar faces. Yet, in the near future there may be difficult decisions to face. What should be done if he gets a chest infection? Should he be admitted to hospital, which is the last thing his wife would want? What should happen when he can no longer take the food so lovingly prepared for him? Should he be fed by a tube? How can he best be cared for at this stage of his life? How can the values of promoting his interests, respecting his personhood, and even at this stage enabling him to live a life as little restricted by the disease as possible, guide the provision of his care?

3.39 NICE has recommended that a palliative care approach, considering a person's "physical, psychological, social and spiritual needs", should be adopted from diagnosis to death, and that people with dementia should have the same access to palliative care services as others.[158] The importance of access to appropriate end of life care for people with dementia has also been emphasised in the English dementia strategy, the Scottish dementia priority paper and the draft

---

[157] Department of Health (2009) *Living Well with Dementia: A national dementia strategy* (London: Department of Health), p53.
[158] NICE/SCIE (2006) *Dementia: Supporting people with dementia and their carers in health and social care*, NICE Clinical Guideline 42 (London: NICE and SCIE), paragraph 1.10.

action plan for Wales,[159] and in the English and Scottish end of life strategies.[160] We have already discussed in paragraphs 3.8 and 3.9 how the concept of 'supportive care' seeks to avoid a sharp distinction between 'active treatment' and 'palliative care' by emphasising the individual's need for ongoing physical, psychological, social and spiritual care, regardless of the existence (or absence) of any form of therapy targeted at the underlying disease. In this section, we will therefore use the term 'palliative care' to refer to the specific care needs which arise at the very end of life. As such, it can be regarded as one component of supportive care.

3.40 As the recommendation from the NICE/SCIE guidelines, cited above, implies, there is a growing awareness of the inadequacy of current palliative care support for people with dementia, and the need to take action to ensure that appropriate services become available. It should be noted that, at present, there is only limited evidence for the effectiveness of traditional palliative care models in dementia.[161] It may be harder to identify when the person with dementia is truly reaching the end of their life;[162] some of the skills involved in providing specialist end of life care to people with dementia may differ from those developed in the context of cancer;[163] moreover, as many people with dementia will already have moved from their own homes into a care home,[164] a further move into the new environment of a hospice would not usually be appropriate.

3.41 Nevertheless, there *is* evidence that people with dementia experience poor care at the end of their lives, with badly controlled pain, little control over the place and manner of their death, and significant stress on their carers.[165] Moreover, recent research in the UK has suggested that amongst older people who die in hospital, those who have dementia are less likely to receive palliative medication, are less likely to have attention paid to their spiritual needs, and are less likely to be referred to palliative care specialists than people who do not have dementia.[166]

3.42 There is further concern that many people with dementia are fed inappropriately through a tube at the end of their lives, without proper consideration being given as to possible alternatives or to the effect on the individual. The National Council for Palliative Care, for example, highlights that current evidence supports "careful hand feeding" as being the feeding method of choice for people with advanced dementia, especially given the benefits of additional human contact and social interaction; and encourages those considering tube feeding to think carefully in each case about what it is that they are hoping to achieve, given the terminal nature of end-stage dementia;

---

[159] Department of Health (2009) *Living Well with Dementia: A national dementia strategy* (London: Department of Health); NHS Scotland (2008) *Mental Health in Scotland: Dementia – A national priority summary paper* (Edinburgh: The Scottish Government); Welsh Assembly Government (2009) *National Dementia Action Plan for Wales*, Consultation Draft (Cardiff: Department for Health and Social Services).

[160] NHS Scotland (2008) *Living and Dying Well: A national action plan for palliative end of life care in Scotland* (Edinburgh: The Scottish Government); Department of Health (2008) *End of Life Care Strategy: Promoting high quality care for all adults at the end of life* (London: Department of Health).

[161] Sampson EL, Ritchie CW, Lai R, Raven PW and Blanchard MR (2005) A systematic review of the scientific evidence for the efficacy of a palliative care approach in advanced dementia *International Psychogeriatrics* **17(1)**: 31–40.

[162] National Council for Palliative Care (2008) *Creative Partnerships: Improving quality of life at the end of life for people with dementia – a compendium* (London: National Council for Palliative Care), p23.

[163] National Council for Palliative Care (2009) *Out of the Shadows: End of life care for people with dementia* (London: National Council for Palliative Care), p8, citing, for example, skills in communicating with people with advanced dementia and managing difficult behaviours.

[164] McCarthy M, Addington-Hall J and Altmann D (1997) The experience of dying with dementia: a retrospective study *International Journal of Geriatric Psychiatry* **12**: 404–9.

[165] See, for example, Sampson EL, Gould V, Lee D and Blanchard MR (2006) Differences in care received by patients with and without dementia who died during acute hospital admission: a retrospective case note study *Age and Ageing* **35**: 187–9; Addington-Hall J, Fakhoury W and McCarthy M (1998) Specialist palliative care in non-malignant disease *Palliative Medicine* **12(6)**: 417–27; National Council for Palliative Care (2009) *Out of the Shadows: End of life care for people with dementia* (London: National Council for Palliative Care).

[166] Sampson EL, Gould V, Lee D and Blanchard MR (2006) Differences in care received by patients with and without dementia who died during acute hospital admission: a retrospective case note study *Age and Ageing* **35**: 187–9.

what the person would have wanted; and what action would genuinely be in the person's best interests.[167] This issue was picked up in the English dementia strategy, which cited a 2004 report of people with dementia dying "with inadequate pain control, with feeding tubes in place, and without the benefits of hospice care", as an example of the need for significant improvement.[168]

3.43 It is clearly imperative that key elements of the palliative care approach – in particular the focus on caring for the 'whole person', the importance of advance care planning (see Chapter 5), the provision of adequate pain relief, the avoidance of inappropriate treatment, and support for family – should be made available in an appropriate way to people who are dying with dementia. One reason put forward as to why people with dementia have traditionally not been able to access hospice care is the simple fear that including people with dementia might overwhelm existing services or make them unaffordable.[169] While this concern may be quite understandable at the level of individual small services struggling to survive on charitable funding, such an attitude within the wider NHS is completely inconsistent with the equal value to be placed on people with dementia and the importance to be placed on consideration of their interests.

3.44 As the 2008 National Audit Office report on end of life care makes clear, palliative care services are increasingly being delivered in a variety of environments outside hospices, including in hospitals, care homes and people's own homes, with palliative care specialists working in partnerships with other health and social care professionals such as GPs and district nurses.[170] It seems highly likely that 'partnership working' of this kind will be the way forward to ensuring that the benefits of specialist palliative care are made available to people with dementia and their families. Indeed, in January 2008 and again in February 2009, the National Council for Palliative Care published practical guidance on developing partnership-based approaches to palliative care for people with dementia, based on a number of case studies and commentaries by professionals from different disciplines.[171] Examples cited include the 'Croydon project', where specialists from St. Christopher's Hospice in London provide both training and supervision within nursing homes to enable nursing home staff to develop palliative care skills; and a partnership between 'Housing 21' supported housing and Macmillan nurses to provide end of life care to a woman with dementia who also had terminal liver cancer and wished to remain in her own extra-care home. In Scotland, the 'Beyond Barriers' project has similarly sought to develop current care practice in care homes by supporting both staff and relatives to meet the palliative care needs of people in the later stages of dementia.[172]

3.45 **We note, and welcome, the fact that the English dementia strategy, the Scottish dementia priority paper, and the draft action plan for Wales all identify end of life care for people with dementia as an important target for improvement, and that the various UK end of life strategies similarly recognise the particular needs of people with dementia. It is clear that a key factor will be the development of models of end of life care which are appropriate to dementia, and we welcome the English dementia strategy's commitment to the development and evaluation of such models. We also strongly agree with the National Council for Palliative Care that close working locally between**

167 National Council for Palliative Care (2009) *Out of the Shadows: End of life care for people with dementia* (London: National Council for Palliative Care), pp19–20.

168 Department of Health (2009) *Living Well with Dementia: A national dementia strategy* (London: Department of Health), p63.

169 National Council for Palliative Care (2009) *Out of the Shadows: End of life care for people with dementia* (London: National Council for Palliative Care), p8.

170 National Audit Office (2008) *End of Life Care* (Norwich: The Stationery Office).

171 National Council for Palliative Care (2008) *Creative Partnerships: Improving quality of life at the end of life for people with dementia – a compendium* (London: National Council for Palliative Care); National Council for Palliative Care (2009) *Out of the Shadows: End of life care for people with dementia* (London: National Council for Palliative Care).

172 Alzheimer Scotland (2009) *Beyond Barriers: Developing a palliative care approach for people in the later stages of dementia – an Alzheimer Scotland partnership project* (Edinburgh: Alzheimer Scotland).

those responsible for dementia care and those responsible for end of life care is absolutely crucial: neither will be fully effective without the other.[173]

3.46 An inevitable aspect of end of life care concerns decisions as to when it may be appropriate *not* to provide a particular treatment for the dying person and how best to manage symptoms, particularly pain, at the very end of life. Such decisions are often difficult, even when there is no real clinical doubt as to the appropriateness of the decision. Staff at the specialist dementia home Vale House, for example, cited the situation when a person with dementia definitively stops eating, and where attempts to encourage continued eating fail, as a particularly difficult ethical dilemma, even though in such circumstances it is widely accepted that tube feeding is not appropriate, and death is inevitable.[174] Professional guidance and literature in this area draw a distinction between feeding difficulties because of dementia, which require a gentle and largely palliative approach, and feeding difficulties caused by other illnesses affecting the person with dementia, which may sometimes require short-term artificial nutritional support.[175]

3.47 We discuss in more detail in Chapter 5 how a person's earlier wishes and decisions about their health care should be considered and balanced with any preferences conveyed (for example through behaviour or gesture) after the person has lost the legal capacity to make such decisions. We note here, however, that our focus on the value of the person with dementia, and the importance of both their autonomy and their well-being, make very clear that a decision to cease active treatment (for example withholding antibiotics that may possibly cure a chest infection) should not be made on the premise that a life with dementia is not worth living. Rather, in such cases, the benefits and burdens of treatment for *this* particular person must be considered.[176]

> **Box 3.19: Example from practice – enabling people to die at home**
>
> In an article published in the *British Medical Journal*,[177] Tim Dartington recounts how Anna, his wife, having been given a diagnosis of Alzheimer's disease, was able to die at home.
>
> Tim was encouraged to write an advance care plan for Anna by her care manager. The plan specified that the intention was to nurse Anna in the family home in the last stages of her illness, as she would have wished. With the support of an Admiral nurse and a palliative care consultant, and the foresight to write an advance care plan, Tim was able to be with Anna "at home when she finally stopped breathing."[178]

> **Box 3.20: Example from practice – enabling people to die in a care home – Sue Ryder Care**
>
> Sue Ryder Neurological Care Centres have set up a programme called Palliative Initiatives in Neurological Care (PINC). PINC has adapted and piloted the three nationally recognised end of life care tools (Gold Standards Framework in Care Homes, Liverpool Care Pathway and Preferred Priorities for Care), and aims to help more residents die in the care setting of their choice, through providing palliative care education and training to Sue Ryder care staff. It also aims to reduce the number of residents who are moved inappropriately to hospital in the last weeks of their life.
>
> **More information:** www.endoflifecareforadults.nhs.uk/eolc/ssuer.htm.

---

[173] National Council for Palliative Care (2009) *Out of the Shadows: End of life care for people with dementia* (London: National Council for Palliative Care), p4.

[174] Working Party fact-finding meeting with Vale House, 30 Sept 2008; NICE/SCIE (2006) *Dementia: Supporting people with dementia and their carers in health and social care*, NICE Clinical Guideline 42 (London: NICE and SCIE), paragraph 1.10.1.4.

[175] Kindell J (2002) *Feeding and swallowing disorders in dementia* (Bicester, UK: Speechmark Publishing Ltd); NICE/SCIE (2006) *Dementia: Supporting people with dementia and their carers in health and social care*, NICE Clinical Guideline 42 (London: NICE and SCIE), paragraph 1.10.1.4.

[176] See also General Medical Council (2009) *End of Life Treatment and Care: Good practice in decision-making – a draft for consultation* (London: General Medical Council).

[177] Dartington T (2008) Dying from dementia: a patient's journey *British Medical Journal* **337**: 931–3.

[178] *Ibid*, 933.

Chapter 4
Dementia and society

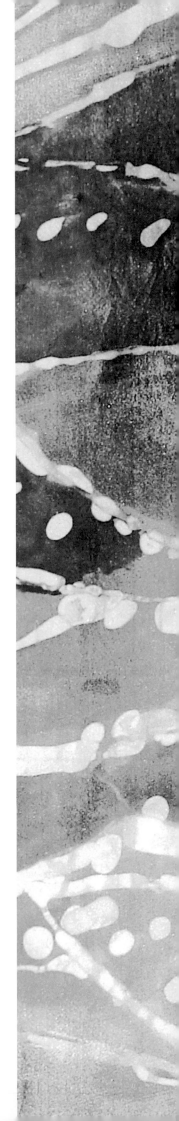

Chapter 4 – Dementia and society

Public perceptions of dementia

> "Even care homes registered for dementia can display remarkable ignorance. I have had families ring to inquire about a room for someone with dementia to be told 'we'll take dementia but not Alzheimer's.'" *Mrs Lesley Perrins, consultation respondent*

> "Alzheimer Scotland is doing some useful work in schools so that children will not be afraid if their grannies or granddads have the illness." *Jan Lethbridge, consultation respondent*

4.1 Dementia is a widely-feared condition, with surveys suggesting that older people, in particular, are more concerned about the possibility of their developing dementia than they are about cancer, heart disease or stroke.[179] It has also traditionally been a taboo subject: in the past people have often been unwilling to acknowledge publicly that a family member had been diagnosed with the condition, or even talk generally about the condition.[180]

4.2 This public silence is beginning to change. There has been considerable press coverage in recent years both of the likely impact, social and financial, of increasing levels of dementia as the population ages, and of the implications for individuals with a diagnosis of dementia. Popular drama series on radio and television have included storylines about dementia. There is regular press coverage about standards of care in care homes, and of the experiences of families in caring for a person with dementia, although bad experiences tend to be seen as more newsworthy than good ones.[181] Well-known people such as Terry Pratchett have done much to publicise dementia by being prepared to talk publicly about their own diagnosis, feelings and experiences.[182] It was also striking that, in our own public deliberative event involving over 50 people with no prior specialist knowledge of dementia, participants commented that people usually felt uncomfortable talking about dementia, yet were not at all inhibited about taking full part in the discussion in the context of our event.[183] This suggested that the remaining taboos may be relatively thin if tackled openly.

4.3 However, it is clear that, although the word 'dementia' is no longer unspoken, it still carries different connotations from most other disorders. As the English Health Secretary, Alan Johnson, pointed out in October 2008, there are parallels with how cancer was regarded in the 1970s: "Thirty years ago, despite its considerable prevalence, cancer was seen as a taboo – an illness that wasn't talked about in polite society and was inevitably fatal … Dementia carries the stigma today

---

[179] See, for example, MetLife Foundation (2006) *Alzheimer's Survey: What America thinks* (New York: MetLife Foundation); Alzheimer's Research Trust (2008) *Dementia: YouGov survey results* (Cambridge: Alzheimer's Research Trust; London: YouGov): in both surveys respondents aged 55 and above said they feared dementia more than cancer, stroke and heart disease. Among younger people, however, cancer was still feared more than dementia.

[180] See, for example, Corner L and Bond J (2004) Being at risk of dementia: fears and anxieties of older adults *Journal of Aging Studies* **18**: 143–55; the criticism of Carol Thatcher when she made public the fact that her mother had developed dementia (see, for example, Pierce A (2008) Carol Thatcher's candour goes too far *Telegraph*, 30 August, available at: www.telegraph.co.uk/comment/columnists/andrewpierce/3561792/Carol-Thatchers-candour-goes-too-far.html); and the initial comments of those taking part in our public deliberative event summarised in Opinion Leader (2008) *Deliberative Workshop on Dementia: A report prepared for the Nuffield Council on Bioethics* (London: Opinion Leader), p11.

[181] See, for example, Daily Mail (8 Dec 2008) *Alzheimer's has made my lovely husband so violent I can't look after him. Why won't the NHS help?*, available at: www.dailymail.co.uk/health/article-1093003/Alzheimers-lovely-husband-violent-I-look--Why-wont-NHS-help.html; The Guardian (17 Mar 2009) *Thousands of dementia patients cared for by untrained staff*, available at: www.guardian.co.uk/society/2009/mar/17/dementia-care-homes; The Telegraph (9 Apr 2009) *Elderly home care patients subjected to shocking neglect – investigation*, available at: www.telegraph.co.uk/health/elderhealth/5124881/Elderly-home-care-patients-subjected-to-shocking-neglect---investigation.html.

[182] See, for example, Alzheimer's Research Trust press release (2008) *Brown meets Pratchett, pledges to rethink funding for Alzheimer's* 26 Nov, available at: www.alzheimers-research.org.uk/news/article.php?type=Press&archive=0&id=326.

[183] Opinion Leader (2008) *Deliberative Workshop on Dementia: A report prepared for the Nuffield Council on Bioethics* (London: Opinion Leader), p11.

that cancer no longer does."[184] Moreover, although reference to dementia in the public domain is now much more common, it does not follow that general understanding of dementia has also improved. In our public deliberative event, it was clear that while people had a broad awareness of the condition and some of the better-known symptoms, they knew little about the causes of the condition, its impact on people's lives and how the disease progresses.[185]

4.4 This combination of good general awareness of the existence of dementia but poor detailed understanding of its causes, progression and implications tends to lead to inaccurate assumptions about the lives and experiences of people with dementia. Such assumptions may serve either to underestimate the effect on the person and the kind of support required – "it's only about not remembering things"[186] – or may encourage wildly inaccurate perceptions about how a person with dementia will behave – "they all get violent, don't they?"[187] There is also little understanding that dementia is a medical disorder and that the symptoms of dementia are the result of physical damage to the brain.

4.5 It is clear that, despite some lessening of the taboos around dementia, and increasing discussion within the media, the general perception both of dementia as a condition and of the lives of people with dementia is overwhelmingly negative. As one respondent put it:

"[There is] a very negative perception of dementia, equating it with decay, shabbiness, and ultimately horror. I say this while reflecting on the response of everyone from taxi-drivers to relatives when I tell them that I am a professor in this subject. People agonise over whether there is a more attractive set of words to describe what happens in my building. But it is getting better." *Professor June Andrews, Director, Dementia Services Development Centre, University of Stirling, consultation respondent*

4.6 At first sight the observation that general impressions of dementia are essentially negative may seem trite: to quote the Joseph Rowntree Foundation, dementia is "not a lifestyle of choice."[188] And yet, we have already highlighted our belief that a good quality of life with dementia *is* possible, for much of the time, and we have noted how people with relatively early-stage dementia have themselves made public how, despite the very serious nature of their diagnosis, they have succeeded in creating something positive for themselves out of their lives.[189]

Stigma

"And whereas no one would trivialise the symptoms of cancer, dementia is an easy target – it is not unknown for people to refer to a dementia sufferer as 'a bit doolally', or 'away with the fairies'." *Speech by Alan Johnson, Secretary of State for Health, 24 October 2008*[190]

"Stigma by proxy is experienced by the workforce caring for people with dementia ... often these roles are not valued in terms of pay." *Admiral Nurses – 'for dementia', consultation respondent*

---

[184] Department of Health (2008) *Speech by Rt Hon Alan Johnson MP, Secretary of State for Health, National Children and Adult Services Conference, 24 October 2008*, available at: www.dh.gov.uk/en/News/Speeches/DH_089682.

[185] Opinion Leader (2008) *Deliberative Workshop on Dementia: Executive summary* (London: Opinion Leader), p3.

[186] Mrs Lesley Perrins, responding to the Working Party's consultation, highlighting the inaccuracy of this view.

[187] *Ibid.*

[188] Joseph Rowntree Foundation, responding to the Working Party's consultation.

[189] See, for example, Joint Dementia Initiative Mutual Support Group (2008) *In the Mists of Memory: A celebration of the circle of life* (Falkirk: Joint Dementia Initiative).

[190] Department of Health (2008) *Speech by Rt Hon Alan Johnson MP, Secretary of State for Health, National Children and Adult Services Conference, 24 October 2008*, available at: www.dh.gov.uk/en/News/Speeches/DH_089682.

"In my experience people have always shown great consideration and compassion towards my wife. This may be partly because in addition to having dementia she is also in a wheelchair because of osteoarthritis." *Mr Keith Chard, consultation respondent*

4.7 One particularly troubling factor about the negative views about dementia that are still widely held is the way such views can lead to people living with dementia (both individuals with dementia and carers) feeling deeply *stigmatised*: as if the disorder were in some way a disgrace or discredit to them. It is striking that, in qualitative research commissioned by the Alzheimer's Society to explore the experiences of people with dementia across a range of issues, the issue of stigma was said to "permeate" many of the responses to the research, even though only one, final, question in the research questionnaire actually related to the topic.[191]

4.8 The Society's research, *Dementia: Out of the shadows*, was accompanied by a detailed literature review which highlighted how the disclosure of a diagnosis of dementia may be seen as allocating the individual to a 'new social group', associated with devaluation, mistreatment, social exclusion, loss of status and loss of friends.[192] Research carried out by the University of Bradford among families of South Asian and Eastern European origin suggested that some ethnic groups may suffer particularly from fear of stigma: traditional spiritual beliefs about the cause and nature of dementia, and associated concerns about the effect of a person's dementia on the marriage prospects of younger family members, were found to be not uncommon in South Asian communities; and there was pressure in both groups studied to 'keep things in the family' and not expose what was seen as private to public scrutiny.[193]

4.9 Personal examples of the experience of stigma cited by the individual participants in *Dementia: Out of the shadows* included unhelpful or dismissive responses from health professionals, with the implication that the person with dementia is beyond any form of help; stereotypical portrayals in the media; and experience of exclusion or rejection in public, with people even crossing the road to avoid a person with dementia. Respondents to our own consultation similarly noted that people with dementia were often avoided, 'talked down' to, or the subject of uneasy humour, while carers felt obliged to justify or explain behaviour to strangers that might otherwise seem unusual or rude.[194] Only a very small minority of respondents stated that they had experienced no sense of stigma and had always felt warmly received,[195] or that dementia was seen as so common these days as to have lost its past sense of stigma.[196] Similar concerns about stigma have been reported in many other studies,[197] and it has been argued, in the wider context of mental health services as a whole, that stigma is the main obstacle to the provision of good care.[198]

4.10 A particularly pernicious aspect of stigma is that it can become internalised: it is clear that many people with dementia *themselves* struggle with a sense of shame and inadequacy and feel 'lesser

---

[191] Alzheimer's Society (2008) *Dementia: Out of the shadows* (London: Alzheimer's Society), p55.

[192] Alzheimer's Society (2008) *Dementia: Out of the shadows* (London: Alzheimer's Society), literature review, pp 38–9, citing Husband HJ (1999) The psychological consequences of learning a diagnosis of dementia: three case examples *Aging & Mental Health* **3(2)**: 179–83 and Katsuno T (2005) Dementia from the inside: how people with early-stage dementia evaluate their quality of life *Ageing & Society* **25**: 197–214.

[193] Mackenzie J (2006) Stigma and dementia: East European and South Asian family carers negotiating stigma in the UK *Dementia* **5**: 233–47.

[194] See, for example, consultation responses from Professor C.G. Swift and Miss Gill Taylor, and the summary of a consultation discussion held by Stockport Dementia Care Training.

[195] Mrs Linda Tolson, responding to the Working Party's consultation.

[196] Professor Martin Raff, responding to the Working Party's consultation.

[197] See, for example, the repeated references to stigma in National Audit Office (2007) *Improving Services and Support for People with Dementia* (London: The Stationery Office), and the outcomes of the project 'Alzheimer100' carried out in the North East of England in 2007, available at: www.dott07.com/go/health/alzheimer-100.

[198] Sartorius N (2007) Stigma and mental health *The Lancet* **370**: 810–1.

people', as if the damage caused to their brain were discreditable or their own fault.[199] Cary Henderson, an American academic with Alzheimer's disease (see also paragraph 1.16), described his anger at being "belittled", "somehow made jokes of" and being treated as "inferior" and recognised that he himself made such judgments about himself: "I feel that way [no good anymore] and I don't want to feel that way."[200] Claire Biernacki, a nurse running day services for people with dementia, commented to us that "the thing people attending the [memory] group most often say in relation to themselves is 'I'm stupid'. So common is this that at the beginning of each session we display a poster that says – 'I may have a poor memory, but I'm not stupid'."[201]

4.11 The impact of stigma should not be underestimated. Concern about how others will respond to the news that a person has been diagnosed with dementia may lead many people to keep quiet about their condition, thus depriving them of possible support from friends and relatives (and indeed possibly jeopardising future relationships because of misunderstood changes in behaviour, missed appointments and failure to recognise people). Fear of the stigma of dementia may lead people to delay seeking a diagnosis in the first place,[202] while offhand, dismissive responses by health professionals can close the doors to more specialist help.[203] Stigma may make it harder still for people to retain their self-esteem and sense of status within society, as they attempt to come to terms with their changing cognitive abilities and sense of self.[204] Moreover, the stigma associated with dementia inevitably has an effect on the status of services and the enthusiasm of professionals and other paid staff to work in them, which in turn may lead to poorer quality care.[205]

4.12 There are many medical conditions, such as serious respiratory or muscular conditions, that, like dementia, can have a major impact on people's lives, but which are not stigmatised in the same way as dementia: the symptoms of such conditions may be feared, but the conditions themselves are not regarded as shameful. The National Audit Office noted in its 2007 report on dementia that a similar attitude to cancer in the 1950s had been transformed by a combination of technological advances, raised awareness and culture change.[206] This comparison with cancer suggests a number of inter-related causes of stigma, including ignorance about the condition and a sense of helplessness in the face of a disease for which there is no ready 'cure', leading to fear and denial.

4.13 An additional and, in the case of dementia, crucial factor is the fact that the physical damage caused to the brain by the underlying disease has a significant and progressive impact on a person's cognitive abilities and their ability to exert control over their own life, both of which can affect a person's self-esteem and sense of self.[207] One person with dementia described her diagnosis as like being "certified as a non-person."[208] Moreover, dementia is predominately a disease of old age, a period in life associated with increasing physical decline, vulnerability and dependence. The discrimination and stigma associated with mental illness, with old age and with increased

---

[199] See, for example, Katsuno T (2005) Dementia from the inside: how people with early-stage dementia evaluate their quality of life *Ageing and Society* **25**: 197–214.

[200] Henderson CS (1998) *Partial View – An Alzheimer's journal* (Dallas: Southern Methodist University Press), pp37 and 82.

[201] Claire Biernacki, responding to the Working Party's consultation.

[202] National Audit Office (2007) *Improving Services and Support for People with Dementia* (London: The Stationery Office), p24.

[203] Age Concern (2008) *Out of Sight, Out of Mind: Social exclusion behind closed doors* (London: Age Concern), p35.

[204] Katsuno T (2005) Dementia from the inside: how people with early-stage dementia evaluate their quality of life *Ageing and Society* **25**: 197–214.

[205] See, for example, consultation responses from June Andrews and Admiral Nurses – 'for dementia'.

[206] National Audit Office (2007) *Improving Services and Support for People with Dementia* (London: The Stationery Office), p48. See also Vernooij-Dassen MJ, Moniz-Cook ED, Woods RT *et al.* (2005) Factors affecting timely recognition and diagnosis of dementia across Europe: from awareness to stigma *International Journal of Geriatric Psychiatry* **20(4)**: 377–86, where it is argued that stigma is less prominent in countries where people with dementia have access to memory clinics and innovative services.

[207] See, for example, Aminzadeh F, Byszewski A, Molnar F and Eisner M (2007) Emotional impact of dementia diagnosis: exploring persons with dementia and caregivers' perspectives *Aging & Mental Health* **11(3)**: 281–90.

[208] Thompsell A (2008) Life worth living *Journal of Dementia Care* **16(6)**: 5.

dependency are well documented.[209] Those who are diagnosed with early-onset dementia may experience additional difficulty because of the perception of dementia as "an old person's disease."[210]

4.14 Finally, many people's perception of dementia relates primarily to the more advanced stages of cognitive decline, or to the more challenging behavioural symptoms. It may not be widely realised how effectively people in the earlier stages of dementia can function independently with a little appropriate support.[211] Ignorance of the condition leads both to inappropriate concern about how the person will behave (for example, assumptions that people with dementia will always be violent), and also to genuine anxiety about how to respond to, and communicate with, someone with dementia. As one consultation respondent put it: "Society does not deal with difference"[212] – and as a person's dementia develops, they may well behave 'differently.'

Inclusion in 'everyday' society

"What is suffered is as much an alienation from the life of society as an alienation from the individual life of the mind." *Professor David A. Jones, consultation respondent*

"I need the opportunities to join in with everyone else but I also need the chance to meet socially with others like me [with dementia]." *Nancy McAdam, consultation respondent*

"The time for a person to cease to participate in everyday community life is when it becomes distressing and fearful for the individual." *Older People and Disability Team, Social Care and Learning Department, Bracknell Forest Council, consultation respondent*

4.15 Issues of stigma and 'difference' lead directly to questions about the inclusion of people with dementia in ordinary life. A diagnosis of dementia may be seen as placing people immediately in an 'other' category, where it is assumed that the person will not be able to participate in ordinary activities. As a result, people with early-stage dementia often find that people doubt their diagnosis: the fact that they are functioning perfectly adequately in society is seen as undermining the idea they have dementia at all. Dr Daphne Wallace, a psychiatrist who was still working at the time she received a personal diagnosis of vascular dementia, described to us how she experienced both these aspects of exclusion: when she told her colleagues about her diagnosis, most reacted with denial, while one took the view that Dr Wallace should instantly stop practising medicine without any consideration of whether or not her professional competence was compromised.[213]

4.16 The issue of social isolation is clearly crucial for all those living with dementia – that is both people with dementia themselves and family members or friends closely involved in caring for them, who often find that their caring responsibilities take over their lives. Indeed, social isolation was found to be one of the five 'key challenges' facing those living with dementia in the 'Alzheimer100' project. This project, which was carried out in 2007 in the North East of England, used interviews, film, diaries and drawing to enable people with dementia and carers to record for themselves the everyday problems they experienced.[214]

---

[209] See, for example, Office of the Deputy Prime Minister (2004) *Mental Health and Social Exclusion: Social exclusion unit report* (London: Office of the Deputy Prime Minister), p24; Age Concern (2007) *Age of Equality? Outlawing age discrimination beyond the workplace* (London: Age Concern), p7.

[210] Alzheimer's Association (2008) *Voices of Alzheimer's Disease* (Chicago: Alzheimer's Association), p10.

[211] Katsuno T (2005) Dementia from the inside: how people with early-stage dementia evaluate their quality of life *Ageing & Society* **25**: 197–214.

[212] Annie Foster, responding to the Working Party's consultation.

[213] The Working Party's fact-finding meeting with people at the front-line of dementia care, 10 July 2008.

[214] See: www.dott07.com/go/health/alzheimer-100; the other four challenges identified were lack of public awareness/stigma; difficulty in navigating support services; tendency of carers and services to be over-protective of people with dementia; and the long hours worked by carers on their own and without support.

4.17 We argued above in Chapter 2 (see paragraph 2.32) that people by their nature are not isolated individuals but rather are embedded in a network of social and family relationships. The ability to create and develop relationships with others is crucial to our well-being, although personal circumstances will clearly vary enormously as to whether those relationships extend very widely or are limited to a small number of close family or friends. There is nothing about dementia that changes this: indeed, the increasing dependency on others which inevitably accompanies dementia emphasises, rather than detracts from, the need for supportive relationships with others. (We will discuss further in Chapter 7 the importance for carers of maintaining their own relationships and social interaction.)

4.18 Clearly the symptoms and behaviours associated with dementia do sometimes affect the *way* a person with dementia engages with others and participates in social events. For example, particular difficult behaviours, such as repeated questioning, shouting or distress, may make it inappropriate for a person to go to a theatre performance.[215] Moreover, some people with dementia may experience anxiety in crowded or unfamiliar surroundings and may prefer to socialise primarily in small groups or on their home territory where they feel safe and comfortable.

4.19 However, such examples should never be used to make the generalisation that people with dementia cannot or should not participate in ordinary activities where they wish to do so. On the contrary, the emphasis in our ethical framework on the value and equality of people with dementia, and the importance of solidarity in responding to the challenges that dementia poses, put the onus on society as a whole to make itself as inclusive as possible towards people with dementia.

4.20 Indeed, we note that this is not only a moral obligation, but also in some circumstances a legal one. The Disability Discrimination Act 1995 requires any "provider of services" to make "reasonable adjustments" to ensure that disabled people may use their services, while public bodies such as the NHS and local authorities have a positive duty to take active steps to promote equality for people with disabilities.[216] However, although the statutory Code of Practice on disabled people's rights of access to services makes clear that the legislation applies to anyone with a "mental impairment which has a substantial and long-term adverse effect on his ability to carry out normal day-to-day activities",[217] the Code itself includes just one passing reference to dementia and gives no examples of good practice with regard to "reasonable adjustments" for people with dementia.[218]

4.21 Good practice guidance on building 'dementia-friendly' environments is becoming available with organisations such as the Dementia Services Development Centre in Stirling,[219] and the Oxford Centre for Sustainable Development,[220] publishing checklists on both interior and exterior design for people with dementia. Indeed, the development of 'dementia-friendly' premises within the NHS is highlighted in the Scottish dementia priority paper,[221] and there is growing interest in the

---

[215] See: Nuffield Council on Bioethics (2009) *Dementia: Ethical issues – summary of public consultation* (London: Nuffield Council on Bioethics), Q7.

[216] ss21 and 49A Disability Discrimination Act 1995.

[217] Disability Rights Commission (2006) *Disability Discrimination Act 1995 Code of Practice: Rights of Access – Services to the public, public authority functions, private clubs and premises* (Norwich: The Stationery Office), p291, available at: www.equalityhumanrights.com/uploaded_files/code_of_practice_rights_of_access.pdf.

[218] *Ibid*, p92.

[219] See, for example, Dementia Service Development Centre, University of Stirling (2007) *Best Practice in Design for People with Dementia* (Stirling: DSDC); Health Facilities Scotland and Dementia Service Development Centre, University of Stirling (2007) *Dementia Design Checklist* (Glasgow: Health Facilities Scotland), available at: www.hfs.scot.nhs.uk/publications/dementia-checklist-v1.pdf. See also the Iris Murdoch building at Stirling University which itself is an example of dementia-friendly design. More information available at: www.dementia.stir.ac.uk/about.

[220] Oxford Centre for Sustainable Development and Housing Corporation (2004) *Neighbourhoods for Life* (Oxford: Oxford Brookes University), available at: www.brookes.ac.uk/schools/be/oisd/sue/wise/resources/Neighbourhoods%20for%20Life%20Checklist.pdf.

[221] NHS Scotland (2008) *Mental Health in Scotland: Dementia – A national priority summary paper* (Edinburgh: The Scottish Government).

importance of environmental design in specialist dementia care environments.[222] However, practical guidance on what reasonable adjustments ordinary service providers such as shops, leisure services and restaurants could be expected to make for people with dementia is not readily available. Yet relatively minor environmental adjustments, such as clearer signage, strong lighting and non-slip, non-reflective flooring, as well as an increase in staff awareness and understanding of dementia, could do much to make services more accessible to people with dementia, particularly in the relatively early stages.[223]

Box 4.1: Example from practice – making services accessible

"One time I was in Falkirk looking to buy a freezer when a seizure came on. I froze. Eventually someone helped me and asked me what I was looking for: I don't know but I'll ken when I see it. They showed me round the shop and when we got to the freezers I said – that's it." *Ross, diagnosed with early-onset dementia at age 52, in an extract from a speech to the Alzheimer Disease International Conference, Istanbul, 2005*

JDI Mutual Support Group (2008) *In the Mists of Memory — A celebration of the circle of life* (Falkirk: Joint Dementia Initiative), p47.

Box 4.2: Example from practice – Scottish Police College Dementia Awareness Workbook

The Scottish Police College has produced a Dementia Awareness Workbook for all members of staff employed by Scottish Police forces. The workbook, which was developed with Alzheimer Scotland and the Dementia Services Development Centre at Stirling University, aims to provide both police officers and civilian staff with general information about dementia; to offer those who go through the workbook an insight into how dementia affects individuals; and to offer assistance in identifying strategies to deal with operational situations that arise involving people with dementia.

The workbook is not a part of the standard training cycle for police officers and civilian staff, and they may choose to go through the workbook – which takes one to one-and-a-half hours to complete – at a time when it is suitable for their individual role.

Scottish Police College homepage: www.tulliallan.police.uk **(Dementia Awareness Workbook not available online).**

4.22 Respondents to our public consultation highlighted many practical ways in which people with dementia could be supported to remain active within their existing networks: these included participation in lunch clubs and coffee mornings, involvement in dancing, art and music, other forms of social events, and continued participation in religious activities. It was clear from the responses that many activities can, with a little imagination, be adapted around the needs of a person with dementia: one respondent, for example, described how she and her mother would slip in at the back of their local church for the last half hour of the service and then stay for coffee afterwards, where they were always made welcome. The person with dementia was thus enabled to participate in the life of the church, even if remaining for the full service was no longer possible. Similarly, while a long theatre performance might not be appropriate for a person who forgets where they are, asks questions or has difficulty sitting still, more *ad hoc* art or music performances in open spaces such as theatre or concert hall foyers would not create the same difficulties; nor would more interactive or café-style activities.

4.23 It should also never be assumed that, just because someone has moved into residential care, they are in some way quite separate from the rest of society. An article in the *Journal of Dementia Care*, for example, highlighted how a woman with dementia living in a care home was taken out dancing every month by her husband: as the husband commented, they were simply continuing the habit of a lifetime, and his wife was still able to take enormous pleasure in dance despite retaining very little cognitive ability.[224] While many people living in residential care, with or without cognitive impairments, find it difficult or impossible to continue their past social activities,[225] some

---

[222] Jones GMM and van der Eerden WJ (2008) Designing care environments for persons with Alzheimer's disease: visuoperceptual considerations *Reviews in Clinical Gerontology* **18(1)**: 13–37; van Hoof J and Kort HSM (2009) Supportive living environments *Dementia* **8(2)**: 293–316.

[223] Blackman T, Mitchell L, Burton E *et al.* (2003) The accessibility of public spaces for people with dementia; a new priority for the 'open city' *Disability & Society* **18(3)**: 357–71.

[224] Lamont J (2008) Remembering the dance *Journal of Dementia Care* **16(2)**: 11.

[225] See, for example, Care Commission and Mental Welfare Commission for Scotland (2009) *Remember, I'm Still Me* (Edinburgh: Mental Welfare Commission for Scotland; Dundee: Care Commission), pp31–5.

care homes nevertheless go out of their way to be part of the local community: for example by hosting local community groups such as mother and toddler groups.[226]

4.24 In practice, it is likely to be the *attitudes* of all concerned (people with dementia themselves, carers, those managing services or running clubs or events, and the general public) that determine the extent to which people with dementia may continue to participate in the activities and social life which they enjoyed before they developed dementia. Two responses to our consultation highlight the very different experiences that are possible, depending on attitude:

"I have no evidence that society perceives dementia in a negative way. We took my parents into restaurants and to the theatre for as long as we could and they were always treated with respect and kindness." *Mrs Linda Tolson, consultation respondent*

"The presence of a person with dementia can stir up quite a lot of anxiety and hostility among other elderly people ... those running these clubs need to stand up to their members ..." *Anonymous consultation respondent*

4.25 More supportive attitudes in society, regarding people with dementia first and foremost as *people*, for whose particular needs adaptations may need to be made just as they are for many other groups, would make it much easier for people with dementia to continue to participate in society. Such attitudes would also reduce the pressure on carers to feel obliged to negotiate access to facilities, or justify behaviour which does not meet other social norms. In turn, increased involvement in society may help to normalise dementia in a way that is long overdue.

Box 4.3: Example from practice – faith communities and dementia

Faith in Elderly People (Leeds) was established in 1982 and works to help community groups and churches to understand and improve the care and inclusion of people with dementia. The group encourages and helps people in the Leeds area to visit parishioners who have dementia, with the aim of raising awareness of the value of older people.

More information: www.opforum.webeden.co.uk/#/faithinelderlypeople/4529885856; **training materials produced by Gaynor Hammond** (gaynor.hammond@northern.org.uk).

The **Caritas Social Action Network (CSAN) Dementia and Spirituality Project** seeks to draw on and build good practice from faith communities in developing awareness of the spiritual and pastoral needs of people with dementia and their carers. It has a particular focus on the Catholic Church and aims to ensure that parishes are communities of understanding which are welcoming to people with dementia and their families. Its work includes the development of training and awareness materials for use with a wide range of people involved in meeting the faith needs of people with dementia, including:

■ People with dementia themselves
■ Carers
■ Staff in residential and nursing care settings
■ Religious orders and Catholic voluntary sector organisations
■ Clergy and parish communities, hospital chaplains
■ Diocesan and deanery advisors
■ Eucharistic ministers

More information: www.catholic-ew.org.uk/ccb/catholic_church/the_bishops_work/social_action_caritas/dementia_and_spirituality_project.

Box 4.4: Example from practice – Dementia Adventure holidays

Dementia Adventure is a registered community interest company, whose staff arrange bespoke holidays for people with dementia and their families. They offer three options:

1. Book a holiday guide/companion to accompany and assist you on your normal holiday.
2. Book from a range of pre-planned holiday breaks that have been selected for knowledgeable, user-friendly services and accommodation.
3. Have a custom-made holiday created to suit a specific set of requirements.

All guides have received education about dementia and have been checked with the Criminal Records Bureau (CRB).

More information at: www.dementiaadventure.co.uk.

---

[226] Ferndale nursing home in Crawley, www.ferndalenursinghome.co.uk/Index.html, personal communication; see also College of Occupational Therapists (2007) *Activity provision – benchmarking good practice in care homes* (London: College of Occupational Therapists) at p13, where the value of community-based activities coming into a care home is emphasised.

4.26 Alongside the importance of inclusion, however, it should also be recognised that most people with dementia clearly value the opportunity to meet, socialise and share experiences with other people in the same position as themselves.[227] The respondents to the Alzheimer's Society research *Dementia: Out of the shadows* strongly emphasised the importance of peer support networks,[228] while one of the proposals emanating from the Alzheimer100 project (see paragraph 4.16) was for social space where people with dementia can talk openly about their experiences and have fun.[229] Age Concern has similarly argued for more befriending projects and support groups, offering "new routes into independence, sociability and well-being" along with "an opportunity to share coping mechanisms."[230] Activities such as 'singing for the brain' seek to meet both needs: providing participation in an activity which is enjoyable and which at the same time enables people facing life with dementia to make new supportive friendships and realise that they are not alone.[231]

Box 4.5: Example from practice – peer support systems

Alzheimer's Society and Alzheimer Scotland

Both the Alzheimer's Society in England, Wales and Northern Ireland, and Alzheimer Scotland work at a local level to help people with dementia and their carers, and many of their local branches provide support groups for people with dementia and for carers. The Alzheimer's Society website hosts an online forum, 'Talking Point', for "anyone affected by dementia."

Alzheimer Scotland: www.alzscot.org/.
Alzheimer's Society: www.alzheimers.org.uk/site/.

The Clive Project

Based in Oxfordshire, The Clive Project works to help younger people with dementia throughout the county, offering one-to-one support services, family support services, social events held throughout the year, and a monthly café for the people with dementia it supports and their families.

More information: www.thecliveproject.org.uk/index.htm.

DASNI (Dementia Advocacy and Support Network International)

DASNI is a worldwide support organisation run by and for people with dementia. It offers peer support for people with dementia and their families through encouraging local groups, internet forums and counselling group sessions, and providing information about dementia organisations in site users' local areas. It also offers twice-daily internet chats, where those who use the website may discuss their experiences with others in a similar position.

More information: www.dasninternational.org/.

4.27 We have focused above on the importance of normalising dementia wherever possible, so that people with a diagnosis of dementia can participate, to the extent that they themselves wish, both in activities which reflect their general interests and in 'dementia-specific' services. However, it is important to go one step further and recognise that people with dementia are not only able (and morally entitled) to participate in the activities of wider society: they are also able to make an active *contribution* to those activities, particularly in the earlier stages of their dementia. One respondent to our consultation highlighted the possibility of people with dementia taking an active role in volunteering, with support available as necessary,[232] while another suggested that day centres providing services and support for people with dementia should be run by participants.[233] One small example of how well this can work in practice can be found in Dorset, where an 86-year-old man with dementia attending a day hospital participated enthusiastically in staff plans to create a 'sensory stairwell', competently undertaking the repainting of the existing wall with only minimal direction and demonstrating clear pride in the outcome.[234] People with early-stage dementia participating in 'town-hall' meetings organised by the American Alzheimer's Association similarly

---

[227] See, for example, Watkins R, Cheston R, Jones K and Gilliard J (2006) 'Coming out' with Alzheimer's disease: changes in awareness during a psychotherapy group for people with dementia *Aging & Mental Health* **10(2)**: 166–76.

[228] Alzheimer's Society (2008) *Dementia: Out of the shadows* (London: Alzheimer's Society), p58.

[229] See: www.dott07.com/go/health/alzheimer-100.

[230] Age Concern (2008) *Out of Sight, Out of Mind: Social exclusion behind closed doors* (London: Age Concern), p36.

[231] See: http://alzheimers.org.uk/singingforthebrain.

[232] Mrs Debra Catton, responding to the Working Party's consultation.

[233] Dr Jeremy Harding, responding to the Working Party's consultation.

[234] Benham L (2008) A sensory stairwell *Journal of Dementia Care* **16(5)**: pp16–7.

emphasised strongly the importance of self-help and advocacy, with one participant commenting: "We can do all sorts of things until our voices fail us, and then the people who are coming behind us will continue to speak for us."[235]

4.28 Guidance issued in 2007 in England by the Department of Health's 'Care Services Improvement Partnership' (CSIP) emphasised the importance of fully involving people with dementia in developing services intended for their use, using a variety of communication methods as appropriate. The guidance also emphasises the distinctions between 'partnership' and 'consultation': while consultation tends to be a one-off event, through questionnaires or focus groups, a commitment to partnership suggests a much more long-term and equal relationship between service providers and users.[236] This partnership approach embodies the value of solidarity we advocated in Chapter 2 (see paragraph 2.45) and we strongly commend the CSIP Guidance.

Box 4.6: Example from practice – partnerships with people with dementia

PROP (People Relying on People Group) is a support group in Doncaster run by and for younger people with dementia and their carers/partners. The group meets on a weekly basis, with the aim of providing meaningful social activity for younger people with dementia, including art and crafts, gardening, relaxation techniques, and beauty therapy. Members of the group also speak at conferences and training events, act as 'change agents' in local services and are involved in staff recruitment.

More information: Department of Health (2005) *User and carer involvement in dementia care,* available at: www.changeagentteam.org.uk/_library/DEMENTIA%20FINAL.doc.

Combating stigma and promoting inclusion: conclusions

4.29 We emphasised in Chapter 2 our belief that a person with dementia is to be valued in exactly the same way as a person without dementia. We also set out the importance of solidarity: of recognising each other as 'fellow-travellers' in life, with mutual duties of support and assistance. These values underpin a clear moral imperative to tackle the stigma which is still pervasive in dementia and which leads not only to difficulties and delays in accessing services but also to exclusion, to a greater or lesser degree, from mainstream society. We note that the English dementia strategy includes as one of its key aims "improving public and professional awareness and understanding of dementia", and states the intention of carrying out a national campaign to challenge misperceptions, emphasising that "a person with dementia is no less a person because they have dementia."[237] The Scottish dementia priority paper and the draft action plan for Wales similarly include commitments on public awareness raising and information.[238] We strongly endorse the emphasis placed on this issue. We also applaud the increasing awareness of the importance of involving people with dementia in developing, and indeed running, services provided by health and social care for their benefit.

4.30 Information and awareness campaigns, however, are only one part of the story. For dementia to be truly normalised, it needs to become an accepted, visible part of our society, in the same way that physical disability is increasingly recognised as part of the norm. People with dementia need to feel comfortable going to a club or a class or out to lunch, participating in the life of a church, or taking part in voluntary work, just as they did earlier in their lives. We highlighted in paragraph 4.20 that those providing "services" to the public (including restaurants, shops, theatres, leisure centres, places of worship and private clubs, as well as public services and public utilities) have

---

[235] Alzheimer's Association (2008) *Voices of Alzheimer's Disease* (Chicago: Alzheimer's Association), p27.

[236] Care Services Improvement Partnership (2007) *Strengthening the Involvement of People with Dementia: A resource for implementation* (London: Department of Health), pp20–1, available at: www.dhcarenetworks.org.uk/_library/Resources/Dementia/ CSIPComment/strengthening-the-involvement-of-people-with-dementia.pdf.

[237] Department of Health (2009) *Living Well with Dementia: A national dementia strategy* (London: Department of Health), pp24–8.

[238] NHS Scotland (2008) *Mental Health in Scotland: Dementia – A national priority summary paper* (Edinburgh: The Scottish Government); Welsh Assembly Government (2009) *National Dementia Action Plan for Wales,* consultation draft (Cardiff: Department for Health and Social Services), pp14–5 and 34.

a legal duty under the Disability Discrimination Act 1995 to make "reasonable adjustments" to enable people with dementia to access those services. However, they will often not realise this, and even if they do, they are unlikely to have sufficient knowledge of dementia to make appropriate adjustments.

4.31 The Equality and Human Rights Commission has a remit to enforce equality law, including the Disability Discrimination Act 1995; to promote good practice with respect to equality and human rights in the public, private and voluntary sector; and to undertake high-profile media campaigns to highlight particular equality issues.[239] It is therefore well-placed to provide the practical guidance required to ensure that people with dementia are able to access services in the same way as anyone else, with or without disabilities.

Recommendation 3: We recommend that the Equality and Human Rights Commission should give particular consideration to the discrimination currently experienced by people with dementia, and take appropriate action to publicise both the legal duties to which all "service-providers" are subject under the Disability Discrimination Act 1995 to ensure equal access to their services by people with dementia, and appropriate ways in which this could be achieved. In addition, the Disability Discrimination Act 1995 Code of Practice should explicitly address dementia with examples of good practice.

The role of society in providing care and support

4.32 We have argued above that we have an ethical obligation to become more inclusive of people with dementia, enabling them to participate in everyday life as much as possible. What additional duties, if any, does the state, and society as a whole, have towards people with dementia and their families?

4.33 At present, the needs of people with dementia are met by a combination of state support, family support and, depending where people live, support from the voluntary sector, such as local Alzheimer's societies, Alzheimer Scotland groups or Age Concern groups. Sometimes, particularly in the earlier stages of dementia, the only source of help will be the family and any local voluntary sector support that happens to be available. Where the person with dementia has their own financial resources, they will be expected to contribute to the cost of most state services, with only NHS services (and, in Scotland only, personal care services) being provided free of charge. 'Social care' services include residential care, where individuals will be expected to pay as much as they can towards the cost of their care themselves, unless their nursing needs are sufficiently acute for them to qualify for 'NHS continuing health care'.[240] In many circumstances this will involve selling their home, a requirement which generated many angry comments in our consultation responses.[241]

4.34 The nature of many of the support services required by people with dementia, such as practical help in the home, assistance with personal care, help with finances, and advocacy, is such that these are classed as 'social' care. This classification has two implications: first, unlike NHS services, they will usually be charged for (with the charge usually being dependent on the person's financial position); and, secondly, the pressure on social services is such that support will often be made available only to those with very high needs. The recent National Audit Office report on dementia services in England highlighted the perversity of a system that is often unable to provide early-stage support, even though such support may contribute significantly to maintaining a person's independence in

---

[239] See: www.equalityhumanrights.com/our-job/what-we-do/.

[240] In England, Scotland and Wales (but not in Northern Ireland at the time of writing) a person may be assessed as having such complex nursing needs that the full cost of their care, including care in a private nursing home, will be met by the NHS.

[241] Nuffield Council on Bioethics (2009) *Dementia: Ethical issues – summary of public consultation* (London: Nuffield Council on Bioethics), Q24.

their own home for much longer.[242] Audit Scotland and the 'Sutherland Review' of free personal and nursing care in Scotland have similarly highlighted difficulties around financial shortfalls for personal and social care and associated geographical variations in eligibility criteria.[243]

4.35 In England, there is an increasing acceptance both that the current system is not delivering adequate services, and that pressures on the system are due to increase considerably as the population ages. In 2006, the independent health policy organisation the King's Fund published its 'Wanless Report', which recommended moving away from the current system of means testing for personal and social care to a 'partnership model.'[244] In such a model, the state would guarantee a minimum level of care, and would then match personal contributions pound for pound up to a 'benchmark' level. Those on low incomes would receive help through the benefits system to meet their personal contributions. Wanless's proposals (which called for improvements in the kind and quality of care provided, as well as in the funding mechanism) would require funding increases in the order of 50 per cent, from £6.2 billion to £9.7 billion in 2004–5 prices.

4.36 In July 2009, the Government published a consultative Green Paper setting out its own vision of a new care and support system in England that would be "fair, simple and affordable for everyone, underpinned by national rights and entitlements but personalised to individual needs."[245] The Green Paper proposes a National Care Service which would guarantee everyone in England:

- Prevention services – the right support to stay independent and well for as long as possible and to delay care needs getting worse.
- National assessment – care needs to be assessed and paid for in the same way across the country.
- Joined-up services – all services to work together smoothly.
- Information and advice – a care system that is easy to understand and navigate.
- Personalised care and support – services based on personal circumstances and need.
- Fair funding – money to be spent wisely and everyone to get some help meeting the high cost of care needs.[246]

The Green Paper also proposes three options for funding the National Care Service:

- 'Partnership', where the Government would pay between a quarter and a third of the cost of care, with individuals funding the remainder;
- 'Insurance', a voluntary scheme where the Government would pay the same proportion as under the partnership approach, and would also make it easier for people to take out insurance to cover care costs; and
- 'Comprehensive', a compulsory scheme where everyone who can afford it would pay into a state insurance scheme at a cost of around £17,000 to £20,000 which would provide free basic care to those who need it.[247]

4.37 Alongside this commitment to creating a new approach to adult social care services, the Department of Health in England has also been piloting the idea of 'individual budgets', with the aim of giving

[242] National Audit Office (2007) *Improving Services and Support for People with Dementia* (London: The Stationery Office), paragraphs 3.13 and 4.8.
[243] Audit Scotland (2008) *A Review of Free Personal and Nursing Care* (Edinburgh: Audit Scotland), p4; Scottish Government (2008) *Independent Review of Free Personal and Nursing Care in Scotland: A report by Lord Sutherland* (Edinburgh: The Scottish Government), pp4–9.
[244] King's Fund (2006) *Securing Good Care for Older People: Taking a long-term view* (London: King's Fund).
[245] HM Government (2009) *Shaping the Future of Care Together* (London: HM Government).
[246] See: HM Government press release (2009) *Government launches the Big Care Debate* 14 July, available at: http://careandsupport.direct.gov.uk/news/2009/07/government-launches-the-big-care-debate/.
[247] HM Government (2009) *Shaping the Future of Care Together* (London: HM Government), p95.

individuals more choice and control over their care. The system of 'direct payments' for social care, where the person needing care has the option of receiving the value of services in the form of a cash payment and then making their own care arrangements, has been in existence for some time throughout the United Kingdom. The idea of 'individual' budgets is to create a more flexible system, where the person knows from the start how much money is available (either from social services alone, or from more integrated funding sources), and then has maximum choice over how it is spent.[248] Similar projects are being developed in Scotland (see Box 3.10) while Northern Ireland is committed to introducing free personal care, as in Scotland.[249] The Welsh Assembly Government has promised to support the expansion of 'direct payments' for care services, while keeping under review the possibility of other forms of individual budgets in the light of the English pilot schemes.[250]

4.38 We do not wish to make specific recommendations that may have significant economic implications, nor recommendations about the precise balance to be maintained between individual, family and state financial contributions to the cost of care. This is because we are not in a position to consider the 'opportunity costs' of any such recommendation. However, we welcome the fact that such a wide-ranging debate is currently taking place and we would like to make the following observations in connection with the particular needs of people with dementia, based on our ethical framework set out in Chapter 2.

4.39 People with dementia experience a number of disadvantages in the current system, especially in the way services are subdivided into 'social' and 'health' services, and indeed they may sometimes get 'lost' between the two systems. Their needs are largely classed as 'social', despite the fact that the direct cause of their highly complex symptoms is progressive damage to the brain, and all the evidence suggests that much more skilled care than is currently generally on offer would significantly enhance the quality of people's lives and promote independent living.[251] Under the current system, this means that support services may only be made available when a crisis has already been reached because of the pressure on social services departments to prioritise those in greatest need.[252] Moreover, the level of 'hidden' dementia, particularly among those living in care homes, means that even where people are in touch with social care systems, their particular needs arising out of their dementia may not be recognised.[253]

4.40 We have already argued in Chapter 2 that dementia is a medical disorder and that the needs arising out of the disorder should therefore be met in just the same way as those arising out of, for example, cancer. We have also argued that people with dementia should be valued in just the same way as people without dementia. It is not acceptable to make people with cancer wait until their support needs have reached a crisis before providing that support and nor should it be regarded as acceptable for people with dementia to wait in this way. Rehabilitative and supportive health services such as physiotherapy, occupational therapy, speech therapy and psychological therapies must be as readily available to people with dementia, as they are to people diagnosed with other serious medical disorders, on the basis of clinical need and efficacy. There should also be serious consideration given to the extent to which some of the traditionally 'social' services provided for

---

[248] Department of Health (2005) *Independence, Well-being and Choice* (Norwich: The Stationery Office); Social Policy Research Unit, University of York and Personal Social Services Research Unit, University of Kent (2009) *The Individual Budgets Pilot Projects: Impact and outcomes for carers* (York: Social Policy Research Unit, University of York; Canterbury: Personal Social Services Research Unit, University of Kent).

[249] Department of Health, Social Services and Public Safety, NI Executive press release (2009) *Minister still committed to introducing free personal care* 18 May, available at: www.northernireland.gov.uk/news/news-dhssps-18052009-minister-still-committed.

[250] Welsh Assembly Government (2007) *A Strategy for Social Services in Wales Over the Next Decade: Fulfilled lives, supportive communities* (Cardiff: Welsh Assembly Government), p23.

[251] All-Party Parliamentary Group on Dementia (2009) *Prepared to Care* (London: Alzheimer's Society), paragraph 28.

[252] National Audit Office (2007) *Improving Services and Support for People with Dementia* (London: The Stationery Office), p43.

[253] See, for example, Alzheimer's Society (2007) *Home from Home* (London: Alzheimer's Society), p7.

people with dementia, especially those relating to personal care and those being provided to people experiencing significant behavioural and psychological symptoms, need skilled nursing and psychological input.

4.41 **The essential ethical point to be made is that the access of people with dementia to the services they need should not be determined by classifications of care. In allocating resources, and in determining standards of care, it should make no difference whether the intervention is classified as 'health' or 'social'.** If the intervention addresses a problem that arises as a result of the disorder then the level of priority given to providing that intervention should be based on the needs of the person and the benefits and the costs of the intervention and not on which service provides it. Any future proposals relating to adult social care services must take this point fully into account, despite the current difficult economic climate.

4.42 The discussion above relates mainly to the duties of the 'state', in terms of the welfare support and services made available through statutory bodies. Individuals obviously contribute to that support through taxation. However, we believe that 'society' has a broader role than simply contributing financially to state activity. In Chapter 2, we put forward the value of 'solidarity' to underpin our approach to dementia, arguing that we have duties to support and help each other and in particular those who cannot readily support themselves.

4.43 We have highlighted above (see paragraphs 4.15–4.25) that one way in which this solidarity can be expressed is through practical steps to promote the social inclusion of people with dementia. A further way in which solidarity can be made real in practice is through the more widespread use of voluntary activity. Organisations such as local Alzheimer's societies, Age Concern groups and Alzheimer Cafés depend on volunteers to run a range of services, including advocacy, befriending and sitting services, and practical domestic help such as shopping, help in the house and gardening. While many individuals may underestimate the potential value of what they can offer or may be unsure how to put themselves forward, specialist national organisations such as Timebank[254] do exist to match those interested in volunteering with organisations which can make use of their particular interests and skills, and emphasise that even just one hour a week can be a valuable contribution.

4.44 It is well recognised that there are a number of factors that may deter, obstruct or delay people who might otherwise volunteer. These include:

■ delays with carrying out Criminal Records Bureau checks;
■ excessive and inappropriate bureaucracy;
■ expenses incurred by volunteers;
■ concern by potential volunteers that they would lose entitlement to benefits;
■ stereotypes about the age and sex of volunteers;
■ risk aversion on the part of organisations that could benefit from volunteers;
■ organisations' insurance policies not covering volunteers; and
■ antipathy towards the use of volunteers in profit-making companies.[255]

The Commission on the Future of Volunteering has recommended that the Government should set up a working party with stakeholders in order to remove any unnecessary or disproportionate obstacles to volunteering,[256] and we warmly endorse this proposal.

[254] See: www.timebank.org.uk/about/connecting_volunteers.php.
[255] Adapted from: The Commission on the Future of Volunteering (2008) *Report of the Commission on the Future of Volunteering and Manifesto for Change* (London: The Commission on the Future of Volunteering); The Cabinet Office (2008) *Volunteering in the Public Services: Health & social care – Baroness Neuberger's review as the Government's Volunteering Champion* (London: The Cabinet Office).
[256] The Commission on the Future of Volunteering (2008) *Report of the Commission on the Future of Volunteering and Manifesto for Change* (London: The Commission on the Future of Volunteering), recommendation 2.2. The Commission is chaired by Baroness Neuberger, the Government's volunteering champion.

> ## Box 4.7: Example from practice – the role of volunteers
>
> **The Evergreen Care Trust**
>
> Based in Stamford, Lincolnshire, the Evergreen Care Trust gives volunteers the opportunity to provide practical assistance to older people – including those with dementia – in the local community.
>
> The Trust offers volunteers the opportunity to befriend older people in the community, provide hospital-to-home support, become a member of the Trust's Clean Team where an older person's living accommodation needs some attention, or help to provide meals for the older person.
>
> **More information:** http://evergreencare.org.uk/.
>
> **Leeds Neighbourhood Network Schemes**
>
> Schemes in the Leeds area, run by and for older people, provide health information and advice to older people in order for them to remain independent and healthy. They provide practical assistance, in the form of support groups, transport to appointments and prescription collection.
>
> **More information:** www.leeds.gov.uk/page.aspx?pageidentifier=3ead6668-e3f7-4c61-ad4c-d433220f5f30.
>
> **Finding out about volunteering opportunities**
>
> The '**Direct Gov**' website provides helpful information about volunteering, along with a link to a volunteering database searchable by postcode and type of activity.
>
> **More information:** www.direct.gov.uk/en/Diol1/DoItOnline/DoItOnlineByCategory/DG_069041.
>
> **Use of volunteers in Dutch dementia care**
>
> At the **Osira Group** of residential and nursing care homes in south west Amsterdam, all of which have specialist dementia care facilities, there are more than 1,000 registered volunteers. An ex-nurse manager is the full-time co-ordinator for this group. There is a 'volunteers' agreement' and compensation for travel costs. Volunteers agree to a dress and behaviour code. They are given the education and support required to do their particular activities and are insured for accidents and legal liabilities during their activities. They support residents in a wide range of activities from art, craft and cultural activities, dancing, cooking, swimming and day trips, to doing their nails, playing games, chatting and reading to them.
>
> **More information:** www.osiragroep.nl/vrijwilligers_401.html **[in Dutch]**.
>
> **Training materials for 'befriending' volunteers**
>
> **Befriending Network Scotland and Alzheimer Scotland** are developing a volunteers' dementia training programme, due to be published in summer 2009. The Dementia Training Toolkit will include materials for befriending co-ordinators to train their volunteers in all aspects of befriending clients with dementia and will contain sections on: understanding dementia and befriending; building relationships; maintaining relationships (for example stimulating memory, life story work, motivating clients); dealing with challenges; and recording and reacting to change.
>
> **More information:** www.befriending.co.uk/news_more.php?id=7.

Chapter 5

Making decisions

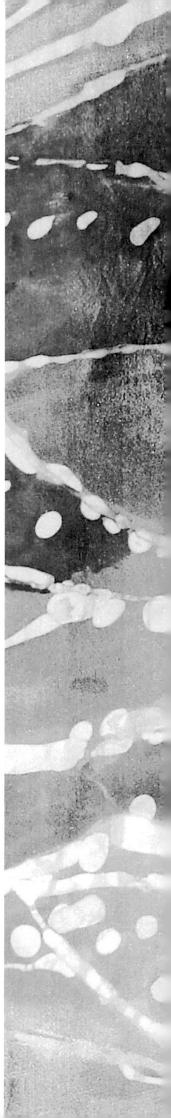

Chapter 5 – Making decisions

Introduction

5.1 It is a long-established legal principle in the United Kingdom that adults who are capable of doing so are entitled to make their own decisions about their health care. In particular, they are entitled to refuse any medical investigation or treatment, even life-saving treatment, and to make choices between different treatment options where these are available. This legal principle applies equally to people with dementia, as long as they retain the capacity to make the decision in question.[257]

5.2 The same general principle also applies to many areas of personal welfare: for example, adults capable of doing so are entitled to decide where they live, what they eat, and how they spend their time, whatever others think of their choices. In making both health and welfare decisions, an adult with legal capacity is thus entitled to make decisions that might be widely perceived as foolish or risky. However, this principle is not absolute: a person does not have the right to demand medical treatments that clinicians regard as inappropriate to the condition, and some treatments may be too expensive for the state to provide. There are also many limitations, based on concern for others, on ideas of what is publicly acceptable, and indeed on what we can afford, that are placed on our ability to live our lives in exactly the way we wish.

5.3 The ethical basis for the right of adults with capacity to refuse interventions, in both the health care and personal welfare field, is widely seen as respect for autonomy in the sense of respect for self-governance: the right to manage and control one's own life. Such an approach tends to emphasise the *individualistic* aspects of autonomy, seeing the person making the decision essentially in isolation, rather than as part of a family or social group where others may have an important part to play in supporting the person making the decision and whose own interests may be affected by that decision. Respect for autonomy in this sense is also closely bound up with the value placed on a person's *rational* abilities, in particular the ability to weigh up options, make a decision, and then take responsibility for the outcome of that decision. Indeed, most accounts of autonomy are firmly founded on the assumption that in order to be an autonomous being, or exercise autonomy, a person must have capacity for rational thought.[258]

5.4 In Chapter 2, however, we proposed a richer concept of autonomy, arguing that it should not be equated simply with the individual's ability to make and communicate rational decisions. Rather, we suggested that a person's autonomy is found also in how they express their sense of self, in their relationships with those important to them, and in their values and preferences. This richer concept, we argued, is more appropriate to people with dementia than the highly individualistic account of autonomy. In order to promote autonomy in this broader sense, we need to support the person with dementia in maintaining their sense of self and expressing their values, even where their rational decision-making abilities have become impaired: for example through enabling and fostering relationships that are important to the person and recognising that people may need assistance in making and exercising their autonomous choices. In this way, it may be possible to help a person with even quite severe cognitive impairment make choices that reflect their values and wishes. In addition, those close to the person may also have an important stake in a particular decision. Compromises reflecting the interests of all involved are a normal part of family life, and respect for autonomy does not mean that one person's interests should always be prioritised over others. This is not simply about balancing one person's autonomy against another's. In the context

---

[257] We do not cover here those exceptional cases where people with dementia can be subject to the provisions of the various mental health statutes in the UK, where the decisions even of people with capacity may, in certain circumstances, be overridden.

[258] See, for example, Beauchamp TL and Childress JF (2009) *Principles of Biomedical Ethics*, 6th Edition (New York and Oxford: Oxford University Press), p101.

of close relationships, what each person wants usually involves taking into account what the others also want.

5.5 We fully endorse the principle that a person with capacity has the right to make their own health and welfare decisions, within the general constraints outlined in paragraph 5.2. The question of capacity, however, is not always straightforward in the context of dementia, and a person with dementia may need care and support from others in order to express and exercise their autonomous wishes. If the person is refusing care or treatment that seems clearly in his or her best interests, and if the person has the capacity to make that decision, then it is important, in respecting the decision, to ensure that the situation is regularly re-assessed. Similarly, when a person has been assessed as lacking legal capacity for a particular decision, it is still crucial to give full consideration to their current values, wishes and feelings.

Legal approaches throughout Europe

5.6 A survey carried out in 2005 by Alzheimer Europe provided a snapshot of legal approaches to consent, capacity and incapacity in over 20 (primarily Western) European countries.[259] The legal systems in all the countries surveyed recognised the right of an individual with capacity to give or withhold consent to treatment,[260] and all were based on the 'presumption of capacity': that is, a person is assumed to have capacity to make their own decisions unless the opposite has been demonstrated. Most countries had explicit provision for some form of substitute decision making, primarily through relatives or court-appointed guardians, and in some countries the legislation allowed for a degree of flexibility in these systems, recognising that capacity may fluctuate or decline over time. A minority of countries have also passed legislation to permit a person to nominate their own decision maker, should they lose capacity in the future, rather than relying on a court decision.

5.7 While comparisons between legal systems must be treated with some caution, since the detail and practical effect of legislation inevitably varies from country to country, there is clearly a broad consensus across Western Europe, and also in North America,[261] that those with dementia have a right to make their own decisions while they retain the capacity to do so, but that some form of substitute decision-making system is also necessary. Thus, although the rest of this Chapter focuses primarily on the legal systems within the United Kingdom, its conclusions may still be of relevance to many other jurisdictions.

The legal framework in the UK: the mental capacity Acts

5.8 The Mental Capacity Act 2005 provides a legal framework for decision making in England and Wales in cases where individuals do not have the capacity to make specific decisions for themselves. The Act was based on the pre-existing common law principle that those who lack capacity to make a particular decision should be treated in their 'best interests', and was developed through a process of careful consideration and review by both the Law Commission and Parliament. The equivalent statute in Scotland is the Adults with Incapacity (Scotland) Act 2000, which had a similar process of gestation to the English/Welsh Act. There is, as yet, no Act governing this area in Northern Ireland, where the common law principle of 'best interests' still applies without a statutory framework.[262]

---

[259] Alzheimer Europe (2005) *Comparative Analysis of Legislation in Europe Relating to the Rights of People with Dementia: Final report* (Luxembourg: Alzheimer Europe).

[260] Subject, of course, to those exceptions where compulsory treatment is given under mental health legislation.

[261] Alzheimer's Association (2005) *Legal Plans: Assisting the person with dementia in planning for the future* (Chicago: Alzheimer's Association).

[262] Guidance issued by the British Medical Association suggests that where an individual lacks capacity, treatment decisions in Northern Ireland will be the responsibility of the treating clinician, on the basis of the person's best interests: BMA (2007) *Withholding and Withdrawing Life-prolonging Medical Treatment* (Oxford: Blackwell Publishing), pp69–70. This is based on the House of Lords case *Re F (mental patient: sterilisation)* [1989] 2 All ER 545.

Legislation for Northern Ireland in this area has, however, been promised by 2011.[263] Both the English/ Welsh and Scottish Acts include a set of 'guiding principles' (see Box 5.1 below). These emphasise the underlying ethos of each Act that a person's ability to make their own decisions should be promoted and supported as much as it is possible to do so. Both Acts also include provision for statutory Codes of Practice in which much more detailed guidance may be provided.[264]

Box 5.1: Guiding principles of the mental capacity Acts

Mental Capacity Act (England and Wales)

■ A person must be assumed to have capacity unless it is established that he lacks capacity.

■ A person is not to be treated as unable to make a decision unless all practicable steps to help him to do so have been taken without success.

■ A person is not to be treated as unable to make a decision merely because he makes an unwise decision.

■ An act done, or decision made, under this Act for or on behalf of a person who lacks capacity must be done, or made, in his best interests.

■ Before the act is done, or the decision is made, regard must be had to whether the purpose for which it is needed can be as effectively achieved in a way that is less restrictive of the person's rights and freedom of action.

s1 Mental Capacity Act 2005

Adults with Incapacity (Scotland) Act

■ **Benefit:** There shall be no intervention in the affairs of an adult who lacks capacity unless the person responsible for authorising or effecting the intervention is satisfied that the intervention will benefit the adult and that such benefit cannot reasonably be achieved without the intervention.

■ **Minimum intervention:** Any such intervention must be the least restrictive option in relation to the freedom of the adult.

■ **Take account of adult's wishes and feelings:** When determining whether an intervention is to be made, account must be taken of the present and past wishes and feelings of the adult.

■ **Consult others:** The views of other relevant people must be taken into account.

■ **Encourage exercise of residual capacity:** The adult must be encouraged to exercise whatever skills he or she has, and to develop new skills.

s1 Adults with Incapacity (Scotland) Act 2000, as summarised in Scottish Government (2007) *Adults with Incapacity (Scotland) Act Code of Practice: For practitioners authorised to carry out medical treatment or research under part 5 of the Act*, 2nd Edition, part 1, available at: www.sehd.scot.nhs.uk/mels/CEL2008_11.pdf.

Proposed principles in Northern Ireland.

■ **Autonomy:** The right of the individual to decide and act on his or her own decisions.

■ **Justice:** Applying the law fairly and equally.

■ **Benefit:** Promoting the health, welfare and safety of the person, whilst having regard to the safety of others.

■ **Least harm:** Acting in a way that minimises the likelihood of harm to the person.

Northern Ireland Department of Health, Social Services and Public Safety (2009) *Legislative Framework for Mental Capacity and Mental Health Legislation in Northern Ireland: A policy consultation document* (Belfast: Northern Ireland Department of Health, Social Services and Public Safety), paragraph 3.1.

5.9 This Chapter will first provide an overview of the current law in the UK governing incapacity and decision making. It will then analyse some of the key ethical difficulties which arise when a person is no longer able to make a particular decision on their own because of dementia, and explore whether, in the context of the ethical framework set out in Chapter 2, further guidance within the current legal framework might be helpful in supporting those responsible for making such decisions.

---

[263] Northern Ireland Department of Health, Social Services and Public Safety (2009) *Legislative Framework for Mental Capacity and Mental Health Legislation in Northern Ireland: A policy consultation document* (Belfast: Northern Ireland Department of Health, Social Services and Public Safety), paragraph 1.4.

[264] Department for Constitutional Affairs (2007) *Mental Capacity Act 2005 Code of Practice* (London: The Stationery Office); Scottish Government (2007) *Adults with Incapacity (Scotland) Act Code of Practice: For practitioners authorised to carry out medical treatment or research under part 5 of the Act*, 2nd Edition; six further Codes of Practice issued under the Adults with Incapacity (Scotland) Act, covering different aspects of the Act, are available at www.scotland.gov.uk/Topics/Justice/law/awi/010408awiwebpubs/cop.

Overview of the legal provisions

Capacity

5.10 Although there are differences in detail between the English/Welsh and Scottish Acts and the proposals in Northern Ireland, in each case the underlying approach to the concept of incapacity is broadly the same. In all three jurisdictions, the starting point is that a person will be presumed to have capacity to make a particular decision unless the contrary is demonstrated. A person will be held to lack legal capacity in connection with a particular decision only if they are incapable of making, understanding or communicating that decision. Capacity should always be 'decision-specific': an individual may lack capacity to make one decision but retain sufficient capacity to make another decision. It may also fluctuate: a person may lack the capacity to make a particular decision in the evening when they are tired, for example, but be quite capable of making the same decision in the morning. Both the English/Welsh and Scottish Acts also specify that all reasonable attempts must be made to help people make their own decisions, and the Northern Ireland proposals similarly state that the "new legislation should support people to make their own decisions."[265]

5.11 These approaches to capacity are particularly important in connection with dementia, where capacity may fluctuate significantly, and where capacity may be retained for some decisions long after it is lost for others. It is to be hoped, therefore, that anecdotal evidence of professionals and care workers mistakenly assuming that incapacity is a general condition, rather than being decision-specific, will quickly become a thing of the past.

Best interests and benefit

5.12 Although the underlying approach to lack of capacity is similar across the UK, the statutory provisions in England/Wales and in Scotland do differ both in terms of language and in the structures and systems used to protect and promote the welfare of those who lack legal capacity.[266] In England and Wales, if an individual lacks capacity to make a particular decision (and has not made a valid and applicable advance decision as described in paragraph 5.15), then the Mental Capacity Act specifies that others, such as family, friends, or health and social care professionals, must act in the individual's 'best interests.'

5.13 There is no simple definition of best interests in the Act, but includes factors that should be considered when judging best interests, including the person's "past and present wishes and feelings", and "the beliefs and values that would be likely to influence his decision if he had capacity" (see Box 5.2 below). Nor does the Act spell out *who* should take particular decisions: rather it states that people act lawfully if they reasonably believe that they are acting in the incapacitated person's best interests.

5.14 In Scotland, the Adults with Incapacity (Scotland) Act does not use the language of 'best interests', and instead requires that any intervention must *benefit* the adult, in a way that could not be achieved without the intervention. When deciding whether an intervention is justified, the Scottish Act suggests that account should be taken of "the present and past wishes and feelings of the adult" and also of the views of those closely involved with the individual.

---

[265] Northern Ireland Department of Health, Social Services and Public Safety (2009) *Legislative Framework for Mental Capacity and Mental Health Legislation in Northern Ireland: A policy consultation document* (Belfast: Northern Ireland Department of Health, Social Services and Public Safety), paragraph 4.1.

[266] The Northern Ireland legislative proposals published in January 2009 do not go into this degree of detail but simply note that the proposed Mental Capacity Bill "will provide detail on what substitute decision makers will need to take account of when acting on behalf of an individual with impaired capacity" – see Northern Ireland Department of Health, Social Services and Public Safety (2009) *Legislative Framework for Mental Capacity and Mental Health Legislation in Northern Ireland: A policy consultation document* (Belfast: Northern Ireland Department of Health, Social Services and Public Safety), paragraph 4.3.

> **Box 5.2: Best interests and benefit**
>
> **'Best interests' in England and Wales**
>
> Factors to take into account when determining a person's best interests include:
>
> - the person's past and present wishes and feelings (in particular any relevant written statements made before loss of capacity);
> - the beliefs and values that would be likely to influence the person's decision if they had capacity;
> - other factors they would be likely to consider if they were able to do so; and
> - where practical and appropriate, the views of a number of others concerned with the person's welfare as to what action would be in the person's best interests.
>
> The person who lacks capacity must be encouraged to participate as fully as possible in any decision taken on their behalf.
> ss4(4), 4(6) and 4(7) Mental Capacity Act 2005.
>
> **'Benefit' in Scotland**
>
> Factors to be taken into account when determining whether an intervention might benefit an adult include:
>
> - the person's past and present wishes and feelings; and
> - the views of a number of others concerned with the person's welfare, in so far as it is reasonable and practicable to obtain them.
>
> The person who lacks capacity must be encouraged to participate as fully as possible in any decision taken on their behalf.
> s1(4) Adults with Incapacity (Scotland) Act 2000.

Advance decisions

5.15 The Mental Capacity Act also makes specific provision for people in England and Wales to make 'advance decisions' to refuse treatment. Such decisions are legally binding on professionals if they are valid and applicable to the treatment in question. They will not, however, be binding if they have been invalidated in some way, for example if people change their mind while they still have capacity, or if they do "anything else clearly inconsistent with the advance decision remaining [their] fixed decision."[267] The Northern Ireland proposals also include provision for advance decisions to refuse treatment.[268] The Adults with Incapacity (Scotland) Act does not make any reference to advance refusals of treatment, although the Scottish Code of Practice notes that they are "potentially binding."[269] Advance decisions are discussed further in paragraphs 5.33–5.49.

Proxy decision making

5.16 Both mental capacity Acts also make provision for 'proxy' decision making. People who still have the capacity to do so may nominate someone, typically a spouse or close relative, to be a 'welfare attorney' to make health or welfare decisions for them in the future.[270] In England and Wales, the legal instrument used to nominate a 'welfare attorney' is called a lasting power of attorney (LPA) and the attorney may also be known as the 'donee' of the LPA.[271] The person retains the right to make their own decisions as long as they are capable of doing so: the welfare attorney only steps in if the person lacks the capacity to make a specific decision. Individuals may choose how much power to give their welfare attorneys: they may choose to restrict the areas in which the attorneys can make decisions, or may specify that the attorneys can take any health or welfare decision on their behalf. The Mental Capacity Act explicitly states that the power granted to an attorney may include the power to refuse life-sustaining treatment, while the Adults with Incapacity (Scotland) Act is silent on this point. While there is currently no equivalent provision in Northern Ireland, the

---

[267] s25(2) Mental Capacity Act 2005.

[268] Northern Ireland Department of Health, Social Services and Public Safety (2009) *Legislative Framework for Mental Capacity and Mental Health Legislation in Northern Ireland: A policy consultation document* (Belfast: Northern Ireland Department of Health, Social Services and Public Safety), paragraph 5.1.

[269] Scottish Government (2007) *Adults with Incapacity (Scotland) Act 2000 Code of Practice: For persons authorised to carry out medical treatment or research under Part 5 of the Act* (Edinburgh: The Scottish Government), paragraph 2.30.

[270] There is, as yet, no equivalent provision in Northern Ireland.

[271] A Lasting Power of Attorney may also be used, separately, to nominate an attorney to make decisions about a person's property and affairs. The rules governing 'welfare' attorneys and 'property and affairs' attorneys differ, and this Chapter is concerned only with the former.

legislative proposals include the intention to create a lasting power of attorney.[272] We discuss proxy decision making further at paragraphs 5.53–5.63.

Review of the implementation of the Mental Capacity Act

5.17 In October 2008, the Office of the Public Guardian (an executive agency of the Ministry of Justice) published a consultation paper seeking views on some of the bureaucratic aspects of the Mental Capacity Act, such as the complexity of the forms used and the level of fees charged.[273] This consultation paper constituted the first stage of a wider review of the implementation of the Act over the following 18 months. Other areas that will be addressed in the future will include the impact of the Act, whether the Code of Practice and other guidance and information on the Act is sufficient, and whether the Office of the Public Guardian is carrying out its supervisory functions appropriately.

Difficulties around borderline and variable capacity

"Perhaps the most important issue is time. People with dementia cannot be rushed into decisions and a structured, clear approach by a person or persons can go a long way towards bringing about a resolution where the affected person is expressing wishes that are not in their family's best interests." *National Prion Clinic, consultation respondent*

"We have noticed that it is too easily assumed by the decision makers in providing care (as well as generally) that people with dementia are incapable of making choices and taking decisions (which will have great impact on their future well-being), thereby 'de-humanising' them." *Christian Council on Ageing; Faith in Elderly People, Leeds, consultation respondents*

5.18 It is well established that the capacity of an individual with dementia may vary considerably in relation to the same decision: people often have 'good' and 'bad' times of the day, and cognitive abilities may also be affected by a range of factors unconnected with their dementia, such as the presence of other illnesses or their current levels of emotional well-being. The Mental Capacity Act Code of Practice highlights the need to choose the best time and best circumstances for assessing a person's capacity,[274] and the Scottish Code of Practice for medical practitioners emphasises that if a decision can be deferred until a time when a person is likely to have sufficient capacity to take it, then it should be.[275] This approach was reiterated by a number of respondents to our consultation. It is also important to note that the *way* a person is approached and spoken to may in itself affect their capacity or apparent capacity to make a decision: it is increasingly recognised how the use of an infantilising manner or language – 'elderspeak' – actively disempowers older people from involvement in their own care.[276]

5.19 However, the assessment of a person's capacity can never be an exact science (particularly where there are significant communication difficulties), and it is still quite possible that different professionals, acting in full knowledge of the Acts, may come to different conclusions as to whether the person

---

[272] Northern Ireland Department of Health, Social Services and Public Safety (2009) *Legislative Framework for Mental Capacity and Mental Health Legislation in Northern Ireland: A policy consultation document* (Belfast: Northern Ireland Department of Health, Social Services and Public Safety), paragraph 5.1.

[273] Office of the Public Guardian (2008) *Reviewing the Mental Capacity Act 2005: Forms, supervision and fees – consultation paper CP26/08* (London: Ministry of Justice).

[274] Department for Constitutional Affairs (2007) *Mental Capacity Act 2005 Code of Practice* (London: The Stationery Office), paragraph 4.36.

[275] Scottish Government (2007) *Adults with Incapacity (Scotland) Act 2000 Code of Practice: For persons authorised to carry out medical treatment or research under Part 5 of the Act* (Edinburgh: The Scottish Government), paragraph 1.16.

[276] See, for example, University of Kansas Medical Center News Release (2008) *Respectful adult communication improves quality of care in Alzheimer's patients*, 28 July, available at: www2.ku.edu/~kugeron/news/; British Medical Association (2009) *The Ethics of Caring for Older People*, 2nd Edition (Chichester: Wiley-Blackwell), pp20–1.

has sufficient understanding to make a particular decision at a particular time. The implications for the individuals concerned are potentially very significant: if they are assessed as having capacity they will be free to choose their own course of action (even if regarded by as others as highly risky), whereas if they are assessed as lacking capacity their wishes may be overruled by others in the hope of protecting their best interests.

5.20 Under the current law, a person either has, or does not have, the capacity to make a particular decision at a particular point in time, and it is difficult to see how else a law could be framed without creating "an impossibly woolly situation."[277] However, as the examples above suggest, this approach is itself problematic with respect to important decisions, particularly in the earlier stages of dementia, where very different outcomes may arise from marginal differences in capacity (or indeed in opinions about capacity).

5.21 One possible approach that has been suggested for avoiding, or at least reducing, the problems inherent in borderline capacity is greater emphasis around joint decision making with trusted family members. It is suggested that such *joint* decision making might help bridge the gap between the time when a person with dementia is fully able to make his or her own decisions, and the time when some kind of formal proxy decision making becomes necessary on a regular basis.[278] Indeed, such an approach is implicit in the requirement set out in both the Mental Capacity Act and the Adults with Incapacity (Scotland) Act that all practicable steps must be taken to help an individual make a decision before concluding that he or she lacks capacity.[279]

5.22 Clearly, it would be important that such an arrangement did not undermine the use of a welfare power of attorney where dementia had progressed to the point that this became necessary. Moreover, the appropriateness of family involvement would always depend heavily on existing family relationships: some people with dementia will have family members whom they trust, and whom professionals also feel able to trust, and others will not. The extent to which the person with dementia is willing to share their confidential clinical information with others will also vary considerably from person to person. However, professionals could facilitate such an approach for those who would welcome it, by making clear from the outset that they are willing to engage and communicate with carers and family members, and facilitate joint decision making, if that is what the person with dementia wishes. We note that such an approach is consistent with our earlier recommendation (see paragraph 3.23) that professionals should encourage people receiving a diagnosis of dementia to share that information with those close to them, on the basis that dementia, more than many other health conditions, affects whole families and not just individuals.

5.23 **As we discuss in Chapter 2, most people do not make 'autonomous' decisions in isolation: rather they come to decisions supported by those close to them and in the light of those relationships (see paragraphs 2.31–2.32). Joint decision making with trusted family or friends is one example of how our broader approach to autonomy can be realised in practice, and is potentially valuable both in meeting the legal requirement to take all practicable steps to support a person in making their own decision and in supporting the person in 'borderline' cases where their capacity is uncertain.**

Recommendation 4: We recommend that the Codes of Practice made under the Mental Capacity Act and the Adults with Incapacity (Scotland) Act should be amended to emphasise the importance of good communication and supportive relationships with families, so that joint decision making is encouraged wherever appropriate.

---

[277] Dr Ian M. Jessiman, responding to the Working Party's consultation.

[278] Nuffield Council on Bioethics (2009) *Dementia: Ethical issues – summary of public consultation* (London: Nuffield Council on Bioethics), Q14; see also Molinari V, McCullough LB, Coverdale JH and Workman R (2006) Principles and practice of geriatric assent *Aging & Mental Health* **10(1)**: 48–54 where an "active collaboration" between health professionals and people with impaired capacity is promoted.

[279] s1(3) Mental Capacity Act 2005; s1(5) Adults with Incapacity (Scotland) Act 2000.

Determining best interests/benefit: balancing past and present

"... if the person expressly requested things when they had capacity, then those wishes should be adhered to." *Daphne Sharp, consultation respondent*

"Preventing someone from taking actions that make them happy now because it may not have made their old selves happy is difficult." *European Care Group, consultation respondent*

"If his/her current wishes and values are totally at odds with the past, then it would be helpful to try to understand the change... whether it is based, for example, on a sense of insecurity, fear or as consequence of the illness e.g. disinhibited behaviour; or because the person is genuinely enjoying doing things differently." *Alzheimer Scotland, consultation respondent*

5.24 Given the central role 'best interests' or 'benefit' play in legal provisions, a crucial question which must be addressed is how these terms should be understood. In Chapter 2, we identified two distinct sets of interests to be considered: on the one hand, a person's 'autonomy interests', which include having the freedom to act in accordance with one's own values, in a way that seems true to oneself; and, on the other, their 'well-being interests', which include both maximising day-to-day happiness and promoting aspects of the person's life which are seen as objectively good. The legal approach to best interests in England/Wales and in Scotland includes consideration of both these sets of interests, requiring decision makers to consider both what would be ordinary good practice in clinical care and what the person in question might have chosen when they had capacity.[280]

5.25 When considering what kind of decision the person would have made, had they still had capacity, the English/Welsh and the Scottish Acts refer to both 'past' and 'present' wishes and feelings. In many cases there will be clear continuity between the way people with dementia approach their life now and in the past. However, situations can and do arise where an individual's past and present views on a particular question seem to diverge sharply. In these circumstances, the Scottish Code of Practice for medical professionals suggests that "the most recently expressed view/wish made while the adult had capacity, will prevail."[281] The English/Welsh Code of Practice is less specific, highlighting the importance of strong views in the past, particularly those set down in writing, but emphasising that these would not be the only factor to take into account when considering best interests.[282]

> **Case example: Mrs A**[283]
>
> Earlier in her life, Mrs A made it clear that she would not value life with dementia and if, at some point in the future, she were to develop dementia and lose capacity to make her own decisions, she would not want any medical treatment which might prolong her life. Mrs A goes on to develop dementia. She appears to be contented, spending her days happily reading random pages of a detective story, enjoying walking round the garden, drawing the same picture repeatedly, and eating her favourite food. Difficulties may arise in determining whether her past or present preferences should dominate when making critical decisions about her health care if she is not able to form or communicate her views herself: for example, whether she should be given antibiotics to treat a chest infection in circumstances where the antibiotics would be highly likely to prolong her life.

---

[280] The Northern Ireland legislative proposals published in January 2009 do not go into this degree of detail but simply note that the proposed Mental Capacity Bill "will provide detail on what substitute decision makers will need to take account of when acting on behalf of an individual with impaired capacity" – see Northern Ireland Department of Health, Social Services and Public Safety (2009) *Legislative Framework for Mental Capacity and Mental Health Legislation in Northern Ireland: A policy consultation document* (Belfast: Northern Ireland Department of Health, Social Services and Public Safety), paragraph 4.3.

[281] Scottish Government (2007) *Adults with Incapacity (Scotland) Act 2000 Code of Practice: For persons authorised to carry out medical treatment or research under Part 5 of the Act* (Edinburgh: The Scottish Government), paragraph 2.33.

[282] Department for Constitutional Affairs (2007) *Mental Capacity Act 2005 Code of Practice* (London: The Stationery Office), paragraphs 5.40–5.

[283] Based on the case of 'Margo' as described in Firlik AD (1991) Margo's logo *Journal of the American Medical Association* **265(2)**: 201.

5.26 As the case of Mrs A demonstrates, it may not always be easy to decide what course of action is genuinely in a person's best interests. There are very strong differences of opinion among ethicists as to whether previously held opinions or current preferences should take precedence in such circumstances,[284] and similarly conflicting views were apparent both in the responses we received from our public consultation questions on this issue,[285] and in our public deliberative event involving members of the public with little or no prior knowledge of dementia.[286] Indeed, it was noticeable that this was the one area of discussion at our deliberative event where no compromise was found to be possible, with participants taking clear and opposing views.

5.27 Arguments in favour of prioritising the person's *past* preferences include the following:

- The belief that such preferences are likely to be carefully thought-through, and reflect the person's whole approach to their life, what they value, and the kind of person they are or would like to be.
- The importance of permitting people to exercise control over their future (incapacitated) lives.
- The belief that the preferences of the person who no longer has capacity do not have the same status as their past preferences, because they cannot be the result of a rational decision-making process.
- The practical difficulties inherent in interpreting the preferences of people who are no longer able to communicate clearly.[287]

5.28 Arguments in favour of prioritising the person's *present* preferences include:

- The belief that a person with dementia, however cognitively impaired, has a perspective that is valid, even though it is rooted in the present moment rather than in the past.
- The belief that people with dementia remain 'valuers' and that cognitive impairment does not prevent people from holding and expressing values, if need be through gesture and facial expression.
- The concern that people should not be 'held to ransom' by their past beliefs and assumptions, especially as such attitudes may change radically when facing major life events. In the same way, people with capacity can and do change their minds throughout their lives, either because of changing perspectives or because of extra information and reassurance provided by others at the time a decision needs to be made, and do not expect to be bound by attitudes and beliefs they once held but have now discarded.
- The belief that, once the individual with dementia can no longer remember their past beliefs and wishes, they are no longer the same 'person' as they once were, and hence should not be bound in any way by those past beliefs.[288]

Our approach to balancing past and present preferences and values

5.29 As we set out in Chapter 2, we take a clear stance on some of these claims. We argue that a person with dementia is essentially the same 'person' as they were before they developed the condition,

---

[284] See, for example, Dworkin R (1994) *Life's Dominion* (New York: Vintage Books), pp218–241; Dresser R (1995) Dworkin on dementia: elegant theory, questionable policy *Hastings Center Report* **25(6)**: 32–8.

[285] Nuffield Council on Bioethics (2009) *Dementia: Ethical issues – summary of public consultation* (London: Nuffield Council on Bioethics), Q13.

[286] Opinion Leader (2008) *Deliberative Workshop on Dementia: A report prepared for the Nuffield Council on Bioethics* (London: Opinion Leader), p4.

[287] See, for example, Dworkin R (1994) *Life's Dominion* (New York: Vintage Books), pp218–41; Michalowski S (2005) Advance refusals of life-sustaining treatment: the relativity of an absolute right *Modern Law Review* **68(6)**: 958–82; Nuffield Council on Bioethics (2009) *Dementia: Ethical issues – summary of public consultation* (London: Nuffield Council on Bioethics), Q13.

[288] See, for example, Kitwood, T (1997) *Dementia Reconsidered: The person comes first* (Buckingham, UK: Open University Press); Jaworska A (1999) Respecting the margins of agency: Alzheimer's patients and the capacity to value *Philosophy & Public Affairs* **28(2)**: 105–38; Dresser R (1995) Dworkin on dementia: elegant theory, questionable policy *Hastings Center Report* **25(6)**: 32–8.

even if many aspects of their behaviour may have changed; that they should be valued in the same way as before (and hence should be entitled to expect that their wishes and preferences should also be taken seriously); and that they remain 'valuers': able to value particular experiences and relationships in a meaningful way even if they are no longer able to rationalise why this is the case.

5.30 However, as we also note in Chapter 2, the person with dementia has interests both in the promotion of their autonomy and in their general well-being. In difficult situations, like that of Mrs A, these interests come into direct conflict. Mrs A has expressed past preferences, in line with her long-standing view of herself, that she would not value life with dementia, and these views must be given serious consideration. Yet, once experiencing dementia, she clearly enjoys and values her life. We believe that *both* sets of preferences should be seen as expressions of Mrs A's autonomy, at different times in her life, and that neither can easily be preferred. In addition, Mrs A's well-being interests need to be taken into account, and her obvious enjoyment of life and lack of distress suggest that her well-being would best be promoted by providing medical treatment that has a good chance of extending her life without undue burdens. Again, however, Mrs A's well-being interests cannot simply take automatic precedence over her past expression of her autonomy interests.

5.31 So how should these conflicting interests be prioritised? Having established that neither autonomy nor well-being interests can automatically take precedence, and that autonomy interests can include current wishes even when the person lacks capacity for the specific decision, we argue that, in each case, it will be a matter of weighing up the relative *strengths* of these claims.[289] Factors which should be taken into account would include:

- How important is the issue at stake? For example, maintaining a person's religious practice or moral beliefs (for example with regard to what they eat) is likely to have been much more important to them than issues of aesthetics, taste, or smartness of dress.
- How much distress or pleasure is it causing now? If maintaining a past belief is causing major distress, then it is likely that the person's current well-being and not their previous autonomy interests should take precedence.
- Consider the underlying values or beliefs on which the earlier preferences were based. Have they genuinely changed or can they be interpreted in a new light? It may be the case that the person is expressing 'old' views or preferences in a different way.
- Explore whether the apparent changes in preferences or values result from psychosocial factors (such as fear) or directly from the dementia (such as sexually disinhibited behaviour), or whether on the other hand they are linked with a genuine pleasure in doing things differently.

5.32 Early (and continuing) discussions on these issues shortly after diagnosis will clearly help both carers and professionals to obtain a greater understanding of the strengths of the beliefs and values held by the person with dementia at that time. This will enable an appropriate balance to be made between potentially conflicting interests if this later becomes necessary.

Recommendation 5: We recommend that the mental capacity Codes of Practice should be amended to provide additional guidance on how past and present wishes and preferences should be taken into account where these appear to conflict. This guidance should emphasise that neither past nor present can automatically take precedence, but that the relative strength of the person's wishes, the degree of importance of the decision, and the amount of distress being caused should all be important factors to consider.

---

[289] Hope T, Eccles J and Slowther A (2009) Best interests, dementia, and the Mental Capacity Act (2005) *Journal of Medical Ethics*, in press.

Advance decisions and advance care planning

5.33 We noted in paragraph 5.15 that the Mental Capacity Act makes provision for an 'advance decision' to refuse treatment, and that such a provision is planned for Northern Ireland. For example, a person might clearly state that if in the future they have dementia and are no longer able to recognise, or hold a conversation with, their close relatives, then they refuse any treatment which might extend their life (such as cardiopulmonary resuscitation) or be invasive in any way (for example, the insertion of a feeding tube). This decision would then be binding in the future, unless the person had clearly changed their mind while they still had capacity, or had done "anything else clearly inconsistent with the advance decision remaining [their] fixed decision" (see paragraph 5.39).

5.34 Advance decisions to refuse treatment, if they are 'valid and applicable', thus take priority over any consideration by family or professionals as to what might be in the person's best interests, and make legal provision, in strictly defined circumstances, for a person's past views to be binding. The scope for making advance refusals of treatment remains controversial, and the arguments surrounding them are based on very similar concerns to those highlighted above in our consideration of how past and present views and interests should be balanced in the determination of a person's best interests (see paragraphs 5.27 and 5.28). On the one hand, it is argued that:

- an advance refusal gives a person control over important aspects of their life (including the right to act in a way which may not be in their own best interests out of altruistic motives) at a time when they would otherwise be completely disempowered;
- such a refusal can stop disputes within families and reduce distress and guilt among family members who would otherwise be forced to make very difficult decisions; and
- it would be a serious abuse of trust not to follow a person's clear directions for their future care.[290]

5.35 On the other hand, it can be argued that:

- a person will not have sufficient information to make decisions for a future situation about which they know very little;
- no-one can predict how their own attitudes may change in the future, especially since important experiences such as serious disease may trigger a re-evaluation of what one values in life;
- advance decisions are unlikely in practice to be useful because of difficulty in applying the decision to the actual circumstances that arise, and because scientific and clinical developments may undermine the rationale for the person's making the treatment decision; and
- it is inappropriate to attempt to bind one's future self in such a specific way, regardless of the interests and preferences of that self.[291]

5.36 These concerns may seem particularly acute in the case of dementia, compared with cases such as coma, where the person's incapacity derives from their unconsciousness, because the person with dementia will retain the ability to feel emotion and experience the outside world, distress and pleasure. Moreover, the stigma of dementia and the fear of a frightening, joyless and undignified existence may lead people, either before diagnosis or shortly afterwards, to make assumptions about their future quality of life that may be significantly inaccurate.

[290] See, for example, Dworkin R (1994) *Life's Dominion* (New York: Vintage Books), pp218–41; Michalowski S (2005) Advance refusals of life-sustaining medical treatment: the relativity of an absolute right *Modern Law Review* **68(6)**: 958–82; Nuffield Council on Bioethics (2009) *Dementia: Ethical issues – summary of public consultation* (London: Nuffield Council on Bioethics), Q17.

[291] See, for example, Dresser R (1995) Dworkin on dementia: elegant theory, questionable policy *Hastings Center Report* **25(6)**: 32–8; Jaworska A (1999) Respecting the margins of agency: Alzheimer's patients and the capacity to value *Philosophy & Public Affairs* **28(2)**: 105–38; Nuffield Council on Bioethics (2009) *Dementia: Ethical issues – summary of public consultation* (London: Nuffield Council on Bioethics), Q17.

5.37 The Mental Capacity Act 2005 attempted to address many of the concerns surrounding advance decisions by requiring that only a 'valid and applicable' advance decision would be legally binding. When professionals are faced with an advance decision refusing treatment that they believe to be in the best interests of the person with dementia, the question of whether the decision is 'valid and applicable' will be crucial. The criteria for validity include such issues as: did the person really make that decision; did they have capacity at the time; were they appropriately informed of the key information (that is, the information that would be required if a person with capacity were to refuse treatment at the time it was offered); and was the decision made voluntarily? Unless the advance decision is created in conditions that provide evidence on these issues, it will be impossible for professionals to know whether the decision is valid; we return to this issue in paragraph 5.41.

5.38 The issue of applicability will also be difficult to judge unless the decision is clearly specified. There may be details of the actual situation that arises that make it unclear whether the advance refusal applies. Consider an advance decision refusing all life-extending treatments when the person has advanced dementia. Suppose the person, in a state of advanced dementia, suffers an acute, life-threatening, allergic reaction to a bee sting. Does the advance decision constitute a valid and applicable refusal of treatment? Since the reaction is life-threatening, on one interpretation it is applicable, but whether this was the kind of situation that the person had in mind to include is not clear. In order to help professionals to carry out the genuine wishes of the person making an advance decision, it will be useful for the decision to include a statement about the values and reasons for the specific refusals of treatment. Such values and reasons will help in judging whether the refusal should apply to the actual situation that arises.

5.39 A further issue around validity arises where there is reason to believe the person may have changed their mind. The Mental Capacity Act provides that an advance decision will not be valid if the person making it has either withdrawn it while they had the capacity to do so or done anything "clearly inconsistent" with the advance decision remaining their fixed decision.[292] The Act does not spell out whether the person with dementia could invalidate their past decision by demonstrating changed attitudes *after* loss of capacity, for example by clearly demonstrating pleasure in life despite having made an advance decision based on a belief that they would find no value in a life with dementia. Academic legal writers have disagreed over this issue,[293] and yet this is clearly a crucial point. If inconsistent behaviour *after* loss of capacity could invalidate an advance decision, this would reassure those who fear that an advance decision could lead to treatment decisions that do not respect the person's subsequent autonomy and well-being interests. However, it would be far from reassuring for those who make an advance decision precisely because they want to control their (incapacitated) future, regardless of how they may experience their lives at that future point in time.

5.40 We recognise that the ability to make binding advance refusals of particular forms of treatment generates very strong feelings on both sides of the debate. While we are concerned that, in some cases, people may complete advance decisions because of the stigma and fear associated with dementia (which we have sought to challenge in this Report), we also recognise that some individuals will still wish to avoid any prolongation of a life with dementia, however good the quality of care provided, or may have a strong wish not to be dependent on others. **If we are to promote people's interests in their own autonomy and well-being, and in particular in their *own***

---

[292] s25(2) Mental Capacity Act 2005.

[293] Michalowski S (2005) Advance refusals of life-sustaining medical treatment: the relativity of an absolute right *Modern Law Review* **68(6)**: 958–82; Maclean AR (2008) Advance directives and the rocky waters of anticipatory decision-making *Medical Law Review* **16**: 1–22; Donnelly M (2009) Best interests, patient participation and the Mental Capacity Act 2005 *Medical Law Review* **17**: 1–29.

notion of what constitutes their own well-being, then it is right that the law should, as at present, permit those who feel so strongly to make those wishes effective.

5.41 **However, we remain concerned that in many cases an advance refusal of treatment may not operate in the way that the person in fact envisaged. We therefore welcome guidance on advance refusals such as that produced by the NHS End of Life Care Programme and the National Council for Palliative Care, which provides a model advance refusal form and suggests a number of helpful safeguards.** These include: encouraging the person completing the form to discuss their wishes and fears with a health professional; encouraging the person to include information about their "hopes, fears and expectations of life", which may help professionals later to determine whether the refusal is applicable in the circumstances or not; and confirming that the refusal does not apply to the offer and provision of basic care, support and comfort.[294] We believe that such guidance may help those who wish to make advance refusals of treatment to formulate their wishes in a way which is more likely to be relevant and applicable at a later stage.

5.42 **We are also concerned about the current lack of consensus as to whether an advance refusal made under the Mental Capacity Act could be invalidated by inconsistent behaviour after loss of capacity to make the decision in question. Such a lack of clarity adds to the concerns on the part both of those who wish to write binding refusals and of health professionals who have to act upon them.**

Recommendation 6: We recommend that the Department of Health should act quickly to provide additional guidance in the Code of Practice on whether advance refusals may be invalidated by inconsistent behaviour *after* the person has lost legal capacity to make the decision in question.

5.43 While we accept that for some people their interests in being able to control their own future are so strong that it is right to permit advance refusals of treatment, we note that the ethical basis for this approach is closer to 'negative' ideas of autonomy ('no interference') than to the richer approach to autonomy which we promoted in Chapter 2. This richer approach emphasises the highly significant role which our relationships with, and dependence on, others play in the development and expression of our autonomy.

5.44 Drawing on our approach to autonomy, we would like to highlight the much broader concept of 'advance care planning' which is now seen as an important part of palliative and end of life care. The End of Life Strategy, published in July 2008 by the Department of Health in England, emphasises the importance of encouraging *all* people who may be approaching the end of their lives to discuss and document their wishes about their care,[295] and the Scottish strategy *Living and Dying Well* similarly emphasises "creating opportunities to explore wishes and choices and help people plan for the future."[296] Such wishes can, of course, include the refusal of particular forms of treatment in particular circumstances. However, they may also include wishes about where the person would prefer to be as they are dying, the people they would most want to have around them and whom they would wish to be consulted about their care, and other aspects of their lives that they find most important and that may help make the end of their life as peaceful and supported as possible.

5.45 Guidance on end of life care for people with dementia published by the National Council for Palliative Care emphasises the need for such discussions to begin early, while the person with

---

[294] NHS End of Life Care Programme and National Council for Palliative Care (2008) *Advance Decisions to Refuse Treatment: A guide for health and social care professionals* (Leicester: NHS End of Life Care Programme; London: National Council for Palliative Care).

[295] Department of Health (2008) *End of Life Care Strategy: Promoting high quality care for all adults at the end of life* (London: Department of Health), p12.

[296] NHS Scotland (2008) *Living and Dying Well: A national action plan for palliative and end of life care in Scotland* (Edinburgh: The Scottish Government), paragraph 23.

dementia has the cognition and language to communicate their wishes more easily.[297] Indeed, in the United States, the development of such 'values histories' is not specifically associated with end of life care: people at any stage of their life are encouraged to think about their values and make them known.[298] This is enshrined in law through the Patient Self-Determination Act 1990, under which institutions such as hospitals, nursing homes and home care agencies are required to alert those using their services to their right under state law to make an advance directive about their future care wishes.[299]

5.46 While future care wishes other than advance refusals are not legally binding, any such clearly documented preferences should be taken seriously into account as part of any assessment of a person's best interests in connection with either their clinical care or general welfare after capacity to make these decisions has been lost. Indeed, in England and Wales, the Mental Capacity Act requires that particular attention must be paid to a person's written wishes when making a best interests judgment, thus suggesting that such wishes are likely to weigh heavily in the scales against any other considerations.[300]

5.47 We note that advance care planning enables a person to express their wishes about the kind of care and support they would prefer to receive at the end of their lives in a more holistic way than through a simple advance refusal of specific treatment. Indeed, a crucial difference is that, whilst advance decisions focus on limiting treatment options, advance care planning allows people to say what they do want and what their overall values are. A second important difference is that advance care planning is an ongoing process, not a decision made at a single time. We commend as an example the American *Five wishes* advance care planning document, which encourages those completing it not only to specify treatment they would or would not wish to receive, but also to highlight their preferences around physical and emotional comfort, their relationships with others, and their concerns for their loved ones.[301] We also note, and welcome, the national guidelines on advance care planning published in 2009 by the Royal College of Physicians and others, which include practical recommendations for the implementation of advance care plans, such as ensuring that they are kept in a special section of the person's medical notes.[302]

5.48 **Where individuals wish to make decisions about their future care, we strongly support the notion that this is best achieved within the broader context of advance care planning.** We suggest that such planning should begin early, and should be regarded as an ongoing process and not as a one-off event, with any documented wishes regularly reviewed. We also highlight the possibility of nominating a 'welfare attorney', as discussed later in this Chapter (see paragraphs 5.53–5.63). Drawing on the concerns we have discussed in this Chapter around how an individual's well-being and autonomy interests, past and present, can best be balanced, we suggest that the moral authority, validity and applicability of any advance decision or advance care plan would be enhanced if the following features were to be included:

[297] The National Council for Palliative Care (2009) *Out of the Shadows: End of life care for people with dementia* (London: The National Council for Palliative Care), p13.

[298] See, for example, the Values History Form produced by the Institute for Ethics at the University of New Mexico Health Sciences Center, available at: http://hsc.unm.edu/ethics/docs/Values_History.doc; guidance issued by United States Department of Veterans' Affairs: Pearlman R, Starks H, Cain K *et al.* (1997) *Your life, Your Choices: Planning for future medical decisions – how to prepare a personalized living will* (Washington: United States Department of Veterans' Affairs), available at: http://www.ethics.va.gov/YLYC/ YLYC_First_edition_20001001.pdf.

[299] US House of Representatives, 101st Congress (1990) Patient Self Determination Act, s2(f); see, for example, www.ascensionhealth.org/ ethics/public/issues/patient_self.asp.

[300] s4(6)(a) of the Mental Capacity Act.

[301] See: www.agingwithdignity.org/catalog/nonprintpdf/Five_Wishes_Final.pdf.

[302] Royal College of Physicians (2009) *Advance Care Planning: National guidelines*, Concise guidance to good practice number 12 (London: Royal College of Physicians).

- the information available to the person writing the advance care plan about their medical condition and its prognosis;
- an acknowledgment of the uncertainty involved in the planning process: uncertainty about the medical prognosis, uncertainty about the availability of innovative new treatment, and uncertainty about how the person writing the plan may view things from a future perspective;
- an expression of care and concern for the well-being of the individual in the future, which may also emphasise the uniquely personal link between the individual now and in the future;
- an expression of care and concern for the welfare of those expected to be close to the individual in the future; and
- a statement of personal beliefs and values, including views about individual issues, personal accounts of life in narrative form, and any understanding of the nature and meaning of that life as a whole.

5.49 A more comprehensive and inclusive model of advance care planning on these lines would acknowledge the unique moral authority of the self while the person still has capacity, and also acknowledge the right of the person as they are 'now' to have the expression of their own, different perspective taken into account in judging what is in their best interests.[303] When providing care we should make every effort to understand the desires, interests and values of people with dementia, especially as the disease reaches its most advanced stage. The voice of the person with severe dementia may be incoherent or muted, but we should do everything possible to interpret, encourage and enhance communication, whether verbal, non-verbal or behavioural, and we should treat all such communications with respect. We should value the views and opinions of people with dementia at all stages in their lives, and from the various, changing perspectives that they experience. Our approach to best interests should be an inclusive one, since the legal validity and moral authority of advance decisions are derived from the survival of the very person who made those decisions in the first place. We should seek to acknowledge and address the values and interests of that surviving person, as expressed in either the past or the present, however difficult a task that may be.

Pressure for assisted suicide and euthanasia

5.50 It is sometimes suggested that if people do not have confidence that they will be able to exert some control over their future health care at the end of life, they may prefer to consider suicide or some form of assisted dying as a way of taking more direct, personal control at an earlier stage in the illness. Some people find dementia particularly difficult to contemplate because of the characteristic effects of dementia on cognitive function, mood, behaviour and social awareness; and others may regard any future life with dementia as representing nothing but a burden to others.[304] As a result, some (including a small minority of those responding to our consultation) argue for a change in the law to allow some form of assisted dying for those with dementia. Professional organisations in the UK such as the British Medical Association strongly oppose the legalisation of assisted dying, for various reasons, including arguing that the ongoing improvement in palliative care allows patients to die with dignity.[305] The Royal College of Nursing, however, announced in July 2009 that on the specific issue of assisted suicide it was moving to a "neutral position… where the College neither supports nor opposes a change in the law to allow assisted suicide."[306]

---

[303] Such an approach is also strongly in line with the spirit of the Mental Capacity Act Code of Practice, which stresses the importance of involving the person 'now' in decisions about their care – see, for example, paragraphs 5.21–4.

[304] See, for example, Baroness Warnock's much publicised comments after an interview in a Church of Scotland magazine: Macadam J (2008) A duty to die? *Life and Work*, October, pp23–5.

[305] British Medical Association (2009) *Assisted Dying: A summary of the BMA's position* (London: BMA), available at: www.bma.org.uk/ethics/end_life_issues/Assisdyingsum.jsp.

[306] Royal College of Nursing press release (2009) *RCN moves to neutral position on assisted suicide* 24 July, available at: www.rcn.org.uk/newsevents/news/article/uk/royal_college_of_nursing_moves_to_neutral_position_on_assisted_suicide.

5.51 One of the components of our ethical framework is the belief that life with dementia can overall be positive. In Chapter 2 we have given our reasons for adopting this position. We recognise, however, that some people, when contemplating their own possible future with dementia, consider such a future, at least at some stage, as worse than death. The interest that people have in their earlier autonomous wishes being respected means that this must be taken seriously in decisions about health care if the person reaches a stage when they no longer have capacity to make health care decisions. Earlier in this Chapter, we discussed the situation where a person's prior wishes and current well-being might clash. Often, however, there will be no such dramatic clash: the person with severe dementia, near the end of life, may have autonomy interests, based on their past values, in not having life-prolonging treatment, and (unlike in the hypothetical case of Mrs A) their current well-being may be quite unclear. In such a situation it might be perfectly appropriate, and legal, for care to be aimed at keeping the person comfortable, but not to take active steps to prolong life where there is good reason to believe that treatment would be regarded as a burden by the person concerned, especially if there is doubt about the effectiveness of the treatment.

5.52 But should society legislate to permit active assisted dying for people with dementia, as a few of our respondents proposed? The present situation in the UK is that both assisted suicide and active euthanasia are illegal even where a person wishing to end their life has full capacity. We believe that in such circumstances it would be quite inappropriate even to start to consider any form of legal assisted dying in connection with dementia.

Proxy decision making

Creation of welfare attorneys

"[Ethical problems include] family conflicts over what is 'best' for the person with dementia; and the level of risk that different family members feel able to tolerate at the expense of the liberty of the person with dementia." *Alzheimer Scotland, consultation respondent*

"In general welfare attorneys are an excellent idea as they are appointed by the individual when they have full mental capacity." *Older People and Disability Team, Social Care and Learning Department, Bracknell Forest Council, consultation respondent*

5.53 We noted above (see paragraph 5.16) that it is now possible in both England and Wales and in Scotland for a person with capacity to nominate a 'welfare attorney' who will be empowered to take health or welfare decisions on their behalf if, in the future, they lose capacity to make those decisions themselves. As with advance decision making, this power enables a person with capacity to exert some control over their own future care, in that it permits them to choose a person, or people, whom they trust to make decisions on their behalf, and, indeed, to choose one person specifically rather than another. A welfare power of attorney is, however, a more flexible arrangement than an advance refusal of treatment, in that the welfare attorney will be able to weigh up all the relevant evidence at the time a decision is needed instead of having to 'second-guess' circumstances in the future.

5.54 It is clear, both from the responses to our consultation and elsewhere, that the possibility of nominating a welfare attorney has been widely welcomed. In its current review of the implementation of the Mental Capacity Act, the Office of the Public Guardian noted that the number of people applying to the Office to register a lasting power of attorney (the term used in the Act for the legal instrument nominating either a welfare attorney or a 'property and affairs' attorney) had significantly exceeded expectation;[307] while the majority of LPAs made to date relate

---

[307] Office of the Public Guardian (2008) *Reviewing the Mental Capacity Act 2005: Forms, supervision and fees – consultation paper CP26/08* (London: Ministry of Justice), p9.

to property and affairs, rather than welfare, this may be because people are still more attuned to the idea of future planning in the financial, rather than welfare, field.[308] There have, however, been well-reported concerns about the complexity of the forms required to create an LPA; the cost of legal advice (which, while not strictly necessary, many people may prefer to take); the bureaucracy involved in 'registering' the power with the Office of the Public Guardian (without which it is ineffective) and the fees charged for this registration (£150 in 2008). In response, the Office of the Public Guardian has consulted on revised, simpler forms, and has proposed a reduced fee of £120. There are also arrangements for exemption or remission of fees for those on low income: people receiving welfare benefits such as Income Support are exempt from the fee, while those whose gross income is between £12,000 and £16,000 a year are entitled to reductions of between 25 and 75 per cent of the full fee.[309]

5.55 **Welfare powers of attorney are a very good way of promoting a person's autonomy interests. Indeed, they have many advantages over an advance decision as they permit decisions to be made in the light of up-to-date knowledge both of the person's clinical needs and the care options available. We therefore welcome all attempts by the Offices of the Public Guardian to make welfare powers of attorney as accessible as possible to anyone who wishes to make one, in terms of ease of completion, level of bureaucracy and cost.**

5.56 **We believe that, in supporting and facilitating decision making on behalf of people who are inherently vulnerable as a result of their declining capacity, welfare powers of attorney represent a 'social good' and that, as such, they should, in principle, be available free of charge for everyone. At the very least, a funding mechanism should be found in order to ensure that when a person is first diagnosed with dementia, they are actively supported in nominating a welfare attorney if they so wish.**

Recommendation 7: We recommend that the Offices of the Public Guardian in England/Wales and in Scotland actively monitor whether the current arrangements are in practice hindering anyone who might wish to benefit from appointing a welfare attorney from doing so, whether because of the cost or because of the complexity of the process. We further recommend that they work with the relevant Departments of Health to explore ways of actively supporting people to appoint a welfare attorney at the point when they receive a diagnosis of dementia.

Relationships between nominated proxies and professionals

"I don't feel that the view of a detached professional should override that of a spouse/ partner/child/parent. How does a spouse etc, live with the feeling that they couldn't protect their loved one when it mattered most? Professionals will move on." *Jan Lethbridge, consultation respondent*

"Health care professionals must surely have precedence over attorneys in health care decisions ..." *Mrs Liz Purcell, consultation respondent*

5.57 Although welfare attorneys have the legal authority to make decisions on behalf of the person who lacks capacity, they do not have complete freedom of action: they are obliged by law to act in the individual's best interests (Mental Capacity Act) or be "satisfied that the intervention will benefit the adult" (Adults with Incapacity (Scotland) Act). This contrasts with the right enjoyed by

---

[308] Between October 2008 and January 2009, the Office of the Public Guardian for England and Wales received 22,000 applications to register property and affairs LPAs and 6,000 applications to register health and welfare LPAs: House of Commons *Hansard*, 20 March 2009, column 1338W, available at: www.publications.parliament.uk/pa/cm200809/cmhansrd/cm090320/text/90320w0001.htm.

[309] See: www.publicguardian.gov.uk/about/exemptions-remissions.htm for more detail. The income considered is that of the person making the power of attorney, not the person being appointed to act as the attorney.

individuals with capacity, to make decisions that appear eccentric or unwise to others, or which, for altruistic purposes, are in fact designed to benefit others rather than the individual concerned.

5.58 While in the vast majority of circumstances the requirement to act in the person's best interests will not be problematic, conflicts may arise in cases where the welfare attorney and health or social care professionals do not agree about the individual's best interests. This could occur in cases where there are different schools of thought about appropriate care, for example in the use of particular drugs to control behaviour that others find challenging. It could also arise because of the very different relationships and types of knowledge involved: while health care professionals are likely to consider best interests primarily from a clinical point of view, informed where possible by knowledge of the individual, welfare attorneys who are also close family members are more likely to consider the person's interests in the context of family relationships and family history. This may include not just the person's characteristics and preferences, but also a strong awareness of the concerns the person would have about the effect of decisions on others in the family circle. Indeed, we have emphasised throughout this Report that, in many of the difficult decisions that arise in dementia, there will be no single 'right' or 'best' answer. It is therefore hardly surprising that those involved in making a decision on behalf of the person with dementia do not always agree.

5.59 In England and Wales, the Mental Capacity Act Code of Practice offers some guidance on what health professionals should do if they disagree with a welfare attorney's decision, suggesting that they should discuss the case with other medical experts or get a formal second opinion before discussing the matter further with the attorney.[310] If agreement still cannot be reached, the Code of Practice suggests that the matter should then go to the Court of Protection. In Scotland, the Adults with Incapacity (Scotland) Act makes provision for a second opinion to be sought from a doctor nominated by the Mental Welfare Commission in the case of disagreement between the attorney and the responsible doctor, with the subsequent possibility of appeal to the Court of Session.[311]

5.60 The strict legal position under the Mental Capacity Act is that health professionals are only able to override the decision of a welfare attorney if they have court authority; or in order to provide immediately necessary treatment while awaiting the advice of a court; or if the person is detained under mental health legislation and is receiving treatment for their mental disorder.[312] Overriding a welfare attorney's decision in other circumstances would potentially incur legal liability. Similarly, in Scotland, a doctor may only go ahead with treatment against the will of the proxy if authorised to do so by the nominated second-opinion doctor, if the treatment is required in an emergency, or if mental health legislation permits.[313]

5.61 In practice, however, it is not clear whether welfare attorneys will feel confident in maintaining their own view as to the best interests of the person lacking capacity, or whether they will feel obliged to defer to professional views of best interests, even where they believe their own knowledge of the person will lead to a better decision. It is also not clear how well professionals understand their own role in cases where their assessment of a person's best interests and that of the person's welfare attorney differs significantly.[314]

5.62 We noted in paragraph 5.53 that one reason why a person might choose to nominate a welfare attorney in case of their future incapacity is in order to exercise some form of control over their future. However, unlike decisions covered by advance refusals of treatment, the person is not

---

[310] Department for Constitutional Affairs (2007) *Mental Capacity Act 2005 Code of Practice* (London: The Stationery Office), paragraph 7.29.
[311] s50 Adults with Incapacity (Scotland) Act.
[312] ss6 and 28 Mental Capacity Act.
[313] s50 Adults with Incapacity (Scotland) Act.
[314] See, for example, the discussion in Wrigley A (2007) Proxy consent: moral authority misconceived *Journal of Medical Ethics* **33**: 527–31, where it is argued that in practice welfare attorneys are in fact no more than advisers.

necessarily trying to specify the *content* of any future decision, but is rather expressing trust in a particular named individual to make a decision on their behalf. While there is some research evidence to suggest that proxies do not always correctly predict what a person would, themselves, choose in a particular situation,[315] for many this may not be the key factor. Just as we suggested in Chapter 3 that the *way* services are provided may be more important than the actual service itself, in the case of proxy decision making the *person* making the decision may in many circumstances be more important to the person nominating the attorney than the decision itself. Thus, for example, more important than the actual content of decisions made for a man with dementia may be that fact that it is his wife who is making them. Equally, in some cases, the choice of a welfare attorney may be important in that *this* particular family member has been chosen in preference to another.

5.63 It would clearly be inappropriate to impose a blanket rule that a welfare attorney (or a welfare attorney who is also a close family member) should always have the final say. People with dementia who lack capacity are potentially highly vulnerable, and cases of possible neglect or abuse should never be overlooked. However, the values outlined in Chapter 2, in particular the importance of a person's autonomy interests (as expressed in this case through their choice of welfare attorney), strongly support the argument that the decisions of a welfare attorney should be decisive, unless health professionals have very serious concerns about the welfare of the person with dementia. Clearly this is not to say that health professionals who are concerned about a decision should not encourage discussion and, where appropriate, a second opinion. However, there should be much clearer advice to both attorneys and health professionals within the Code of Practice as to the authority vested in the welfare attorney.

Recommendation 8: We recommend that the Codes of Practice both for England/Wales and for Scotland should explicitly address the question of *when* it is appropriate for professionals to seek to override the decision of a nominated welfare attorney by approaching the Court of Protection, the Mental Welfare Commission or the Court of Session. Both professionals and welfare attorneys would then be clear as to their respective positions. Our view is that significant weight should be placed on the fact that the person on whose behalf the decision is being taken has actively chosen, in the past, to trust the welfare attorney to act on their behalf. This would suggest that others should seek to intervene only if they have grave concerns about the welfare of the incapacitated person, and not simply because they themselves take a different view of best interests.

How well are the Acts working?

5.64 In general, the evidence we received about the provisions of the Mental Capacity Act 2005 and the Adults with Incapacity (Scotland) Act 2000 was very positive.[316] It was felt that the underlying approach to capacity – the presumption of capacity, the emphasis that capacity is decision-specific, and the awareness that capacity is not static – was empowering for individuals with dementia; that the Act had created a clear structure for decision making, which could be very helpful, especially where there was a lack of agreement within the family; and that the status of advance care planning had been enhanced, with the possibility of nominating a future decision maker through a welfare attorney being very popular.

---

[315] Ditto PH, Danks JH, Smucker WD *et al.* (2001) Advance directives as acts of communication *Archives of Internal Medicine* **161**: 421–30; Moorman SM, Hauser RM and Carr D (2009) Do older adults know their spouses' end-of-life treatment preferences? *Research on Aging* **31(4)**: 463–91.

[316] Nuffield Council on Bioethics (2009) *Dementia: Ethical issues – summary of public consultation* (London: Nuffield Council on Bioethics), Q18; The Working Party's fact-finding meeting with people on the front-line of dementia care, 10 July 2008.

5.65 While there were few challenges to the general principles of either Act, there were specific concerns about how they functioned in practice. Some felt that the bureaucracy involved was excessive, with the consequent risk that non-urgent but potentially beneficial treatment might not be given: it was suggested, for example, that flu vaccines were not given in some Scottish care homes because of the paperwork involved.[317] A number of respondents, particularly people working in health care, expressed concern about lack of knowledge and training, noting, for example, that some people working in the field still did not realise that capacity was decision-specific, and that without the right training and protocols staff may "make superficial and inadequate assessments of capacity."[318]

5.66 More generally, there is still some concern from Working Party members' own experience that even though the mental capacity Acts have the 'best interests' or 'benefit' of the person at their heart, there is a risk that, in practice, a 'tick-box' culture may lead to the routine acceptance of unimaginative and unsympathetic decisions about that person's care. **We argue in Chapter 2 that the difficult ethical problems which often arise in dementia do not lend themselves to formulaic answers, and that indeed there will often be no straightforward 'right' or 'best' answer. The approach to 'best interests' and 'benefit' set out in the mental capacity legislation and Codes of Practice is very helpful, in that it encourages a flexible approach to decision making that looks at the individuals and circumstances involved in each particular case. We reiterate here the fundamental importance of approaching such decisions not only with flexibility, but with compassion, founded on respect for the value of the person with dementia.**

---

[317] Christian Medical Fellowship, responding to the Working Party's consultation.
[318] British Geriatrics Society, responding to the Working Party's consultation.

Chapter 6
Dilemmas in care

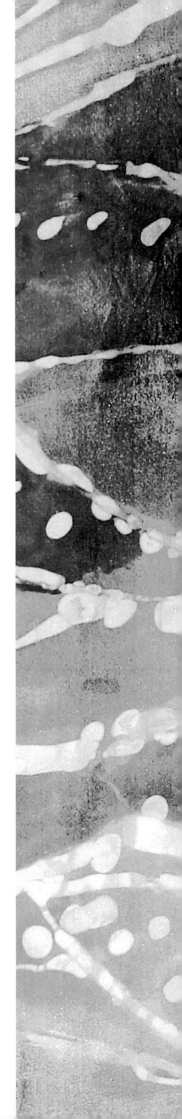

Chapter 6 – Dilemmas in care

Introduction

6.1 In Chapter 3 we considered what an ethical approach to care would look like, with a particular focus on general standards of care. In this Chapter, we consider in more detail some of the ethical dilemmas often faced by those who provide direct care to people with dementia.[319] These include whether it can be acceptable not to tell the truth; whether any form of restraint is permissible; and how freedom of action can be balanced with the need to protect the person with dementia from harm. Those facing these difficult decisions include carers, professionals and care workers, both supporting people in their own homes and working in hospitals, and residential and day care settings. The range of circumstances and different environments in which ethical questions can arise is therefore very wide. There are also many different reasons why such questions arise, including decreasing levels of capacity, changes in behaviour and mood in the person with dementia, and increased vulnerability owing to memory problems, disorientation and physical frailty.

Overview of our approach

6.2 Before discussing some examples of the individual situations and issues that give rise to ethical dilemmas we will summarise our general approach, building on our earlier discussion of approaching ethical decisions (see paragraphs 2.11 and 2.12, and Box 2.1). We consider that:

- Ethical problems arise frequently in the day-to-day care of people with dementia.
- These problems, although arising in mundane, ordinary situations, may nonetheless be problematic and stressful for those providing care.
- Many people providing care feel isolated and unsupported in making these ethical decisions.
- There is rarely one over-arching ethical value that can be used to solve an ethical problem. Critical judgment is needed. Thus, for example, although it will normally be right to tell the truth or to allow people the freedom to walk where and when they wish, there are situations where these general principles are challenged by other ethical considerations such as concerns for a person's well-being and safety or the safety of others.
- As we discuss in Chapter 2 (see paragraphs 2.7–2.12), judgment has to be applied in the light of the particular context and the details of the situation. For example, it may be wrong to tell only a partial truth in one situation but right in another similar situation because of a small but crucial difference in the context in which the decision takes place.
- There is rarely a single right answer to what should be done. There can be reasonable disagreement. Carers may quite reasonably come to different views, one from another, even where the circumstances are very similar.

6.3 As a result of these characteristics of the day-to-day ethical problems that professionals, care workers and carers may all face, our general conclusions are as follows:

1. **Specific guidelines, rules and laws have a particular but limited role to play: they may help to set a framework, pointing to ways in which ethical problems may be resolved, but they can rarely provide a definitive answer to a specific dilemma. Any such guidelines will need to be interpreted in a flexible and compassionate way when applied to a specific situation, with a focus both on the interests of the individual with dementia and on the interests of others directly concerned.**

---

[319] Baldwin C, Hope T, Hughes JC, Jacoby R and Ziebland S (2004) Ethics and dementia: the experience of family carers *Progress in Neurology and Psychiatry* **8**: 24–8.

2. Professionals are in a position to support both carers and care workers, in addition to facing ethical problems themselves. They should have access to ongoing education to help them in both these roles. Education in ethical decision making, however, should not be limited to those with 'professional' roles: care workers are required to respond to ethical problems as part of their daily work, and should have access to the ongoing education needed to equip them to respond appropriately.

3. All those involved in direct care – carers, care workers, health and social care professionals, and volunteers – should have access to forums for sharing and receiving support in making ethical decisions. Carers and volunteers who wish to access more formal courses in ethical decision making should be able to do so.

Recommendation 9: We recommend that the UK Departments of Health consider, as part of their dementia strategies and workforce planning, how all those involved in direct care of people with dementia can access appropriate education and support in ethical decision making.

Box 6.1: Example from practice – ongoing education and support relating to ethical problems

The **Bradford Dementia Group**'s programme 'Cornerstones of Person-centred Dementia Care' is suitable for mixed staff groups, including care managers, nurses, therapists and support workers. The course lasts for three days, of which the third focuses on ethical problems:

Day 1: Dementia explained: the enriched model of dementia

Day 2: Therapies and interventions in dementia care

Day 3: Making difficult decisions: an ethical framework

More information: www.brad.ac.uk/acad/health/bdg/dcm/courses/cornerstone.php.

The **University of Stirling** runs two workplace training courses: one for health care assistants in hospitals, and one for care workers in care homes. Topics covered in both include "seeing the person with dementia", "communication and behaviour" and "support for the person with dementia, family and carers." Ethical quandaries are highlighted throughout the materials: for example, how do you help someone appropriately with hygiene if they refuse to have a bath? Both courses are delivered through a facilitator from the same workplace (supported by staff from the University of Stirling), with the aim of encouraging close links between the learning from the course and day-to-day practice.

More information: www.dementia.stir.ac.uk/pdffolder/Training-HCA-CourseFlyer.pdf and www.dementia.stir.ac.uk/pdffolder/Training-CHA-CourseLeaflet.pdf.

The organisation **'for dementia'** provides a six-month training programme aiming to enhance the skills of those caring for people with dementia, including care assistants, home care workers and nursing assistants. Components include person-centred care, enabling approaches to activities of daily living, and communicating with people with dementia. This accredited programme is also offered by the Dementia Services Development Centre Wales at Bangor University. One day courses for professionals offered by 'for dementia' include person-centred communication, working with unusual behaviour, safeguarding vulnerable adults, and older people and sexuality.

More information: www.fordementia.org.uk/what-we-do/learning-partnerships-and-training/accredited-programs/.

In **Vale House**, Oxford, staff forums and handover sessions at the end of a shift are an important part of ordinary working practice. They provide a regular forum in which difficult situations arising in the home may be discussed with other colleagues, and staff can be supported in responding appropriately.

More information: www.valehouse.org.uk/.

6.4 In the remainder of this Chapter we will describe some of the situations highlighted in our consultation process that pose ethical challenges for all those involved in providing care for people with dementia, and suggest values and approaches that might be used in responding to them.[320]

Ethical dilemmas

The use of assistive technologies

"I have a tilt monitor in case I collapse and a bed monitor that alerts my wife when I have a seizure. All these devices give reassurance to my wife and family." *Ross Campbell, consultation respondent*

---

[320] Further practical guidance can be found in, for example, Baldwin C, Hope T, Hughes JC, Jacoby R and Ziebland S (2005) *Making Difficult Decisions: The experience of caring for someone with dementia* (London: Alzheimer's Society) and Hughes JC and Baldwin C (2006) *Ethical Issues in Dementia Care: Making difficult decisions* (London: Jessica Kingsley Publishers).

"It makes for a better, fuller life all round for carer and sufferer." *Margaret Barbour, consultation respondent*

"How would a confused person react to a disembodied voice from the wall asking why they are opening the door?!" *Age Concern Leeds, consultation respondent*

6.5 New technologies have the potential to make a significant difference both to people with dementia and to their family and friends who provide them with care and support. Examples include the following:

- ■ **'Smart' homes** incorporate a range of technologies in order to react to the movements and activities of the person with dementia in their own home. They may include features such as automatic lighting to guide the person with dementia to the bathroom at night, automatic cut offs for taps and cookers, and presence infrared (PIR) sensors and audio prompts, such as voices instructing or reminding the person with dementia to do something.
- ■ **Telecare** uses remote technology to monitor the health of the person and alerts an appropriate person (such as a carer sleeping in a different room or a central monitoring service) where necessary.
- ■ **Monitoring and tracking devices** may be worn by the person with dementia, so that an alarm is sounded if the person moves away from a designated safe area, or so that the person's exact location can be identified if they get lost.[321]
- ■ **Memory aids** include technological devices such as audio recordings that provide the person with reminder messages, such as "take your keys", or "lock the door." More sophisticated memory aids are being developed, such as cameras which automatically take hundreds of photographs a day, and which appear to stimulate the person's memory of the events of the day.[322] Other devices may be aimed more at emotional well-being, with the use of reminiscence aids, such as those provided through the CIRCA (Computer Interactive Reminiscence and Conversation Aid) project.[323]

6.6 As these descriptions make clear, technology may play an important role in enhancing the lives of people with dementia and those who care for them. As health information and communication technologies develop, their use and usefulness is likely to increase. Devices such as memory prompts may help supplement the person's cognitive abilities and minimise the effect of dementia on their day-to-day lives. Other technologies, such as those involved in smart homes and tracking devices, may enable people with dementia to live more freely and independently for longer, by limiting and controlling potential risks without the need for constant physical intrusion in their homes by others.[324] These technologies may also be of significant benefit to carers in terms of reassurance as to the well-being and state of health of the person for whom they care. The importance of such reassurance should not be underestimated, partly in terms of reduced anxiety and hence improved quality of life for carers, and partly because of the likelihood that this in turn may enable carers to continue providing care and support for their family member for longer.

6.7 In our ethical framework, set out in Chapter 2 of this Report, we started from the assumption that, with good care, it is possible for people to 'live well' with dementia. We then highlighted

---

[321] See, for example, Mental Welfare Commission for Scotland (2007) *Safe to wander?* (Edinburgh: Mental Welfare Commission for Scotland); Miskelly F (2005) Electronic tracking of patients with dementia and wandering using mobile phone technology *Age and Ageing* **34**: 497–518.

[322] See, for example, Berry EL, Hampshire A, Rowe J *et al.* (2009) The neural basis of effective memory therapy in a patient with limbic encephalitis *Journal of Neurology, Neurosurgery, and Psychiatry*, published online 13 Mar 2009.

[323] CIRCA (Computer Interactive Reminiscence and Conversation Aid) Project, available at: www.computing.dundee.ac.uk/projects/circa/.

[324] Martin S, Nugent C, Wallace J *et al.* (2007) Using context awareness within the 'smart home' environment to support social care for adults with dementia *Technology and Disability* **19**: 143–52.

the importance of a number of factors which will be crucial in achieving that aim: first, the need to support people with dementia in a way which will enhance both their well-being and their autonomy; and, secondly, the need to consider the interests of others involved, particularly family and friends who are carers.

6.8 It is clear that technological devices of various types have the capacity to contribute to a person's autonomy and well-being interests. However, use of technology in these ways also has the capacity to act in ways which go *against* these interests. Concerns raised by consultation respondents about the use of assistive technologies in caring for people with dementia were mainly related to privacy, stigma (particularly with reference to tracking devices), and the worry that the use of such technology would replace, rather than be in addition to, valuable human care.[325] All these issues have the potential to affect both a person's autonomy (for example through feeling controlled, being under surveillance or feeling devalued) and their well-being (for example through impoverished human relationships).[326]

6.9 It should, however, be noted that it is not so much the technologies themselves that have the potential either to promote or to harm people's interests, as the manner in which they are used.[327] A monitoring device which alerts care workers that a person with dementia is moving out of a safe area of a care home may trigger very different responses. On the one hand, the person might be firmly taken back to their chair and encouraged to keep still. On the other, the care worker might respond by seeking to find out what the person wishes to do, and doing their best to assist them in achieving it. In the first case, the device may be keeping a person safe, but only by prompting restrictive action. In the second case, the device has not only kept the person safe but has also prompted support to enable the person to carry out their autonomous wishes. Even in this second, 'benign' scenario, it should be emphasised that the technological device is not a substitute for good care: rather it has the potential to *enhance* the care which the care worker is able to offer.

6.10 The involvement of the person with dementia in choosing or rejecting particular forms of technology is also critical. Where a person actively decides or agrees that a particular form of surveillance device will enable them to live an easier or more fulfilling life, that decision enhances their autonomy. Where a person has such a device imposed on them, either for the convenience of others or because they are seen as being incapable of being involved in the choice, then there is a far greater risk that their autonomy will be undermined. In practice, this suggests both that early discussion about the possibilities of using technology in everyday life is beneficial, and that those proposing such technology (whether carers, professionals or care workers) should do their very best to involve the person in the decision in whatever way is possible or appropriate.

6.11 Technology clearly has a potential role to play in supporting people with dementia and their carers to have a better quality of life, as long as the scope and limitations of any particular device are well-understood. Where the person with dementia has the capacity to choose for themselves whether to accept or refuse a particular technology, their decision should be respected. Where the person does not have capacity to make the decision, their own autonomy and well-being, along with the interests of any carers involved, must be carefully considered when coming to a decision about the appropriate use of any device or system.

---

[325] See, for example, Nuffield Council on Bioethics (2009) *Dementia: Ethical issues – summary of public consultation* (London: Nuffield Council on Bioethics), Q23; Hughes JC, Newby J, Louw SJ, Campbell G and Hutton JL (2008) Ethical issues and tagging in dementia: a survey *Journal of Ethics in Mental Health* **3(1)**: 1–6.

[326] Morris C (2004) Personal construct psychology and person-centred care, in *Care-Giving in Dementia: Research and applications*, Volume 3, Jones GMM and Miesen BML (Editors) (Hove: Brunner-Routledge), p67.

[327] Welsh S, Hassiotis A, O'Mahoney G and Deahl M (2003) Big Brother is watching you – the ethical implications of electronic surveillance measures in the elderly with dementia and in adults with learning difficulties *Aging and Mental Health* **7(5)**: 372–5.

6.12 Where a person with dementia lacks the capacity to decide for themselves whether to make use of a particular technology, the relative strength of a number of factors should be considered on a case-by-case basis, including:

■ the person's own views and concerns, past and present, for example about privacy;
■ the actual benefit which is likely to be achieved through using the device;
■ the extent to which carers' interests may be affected, for example where they would otherwise have to search for the person with dementia in the streets at night; and
■ the dangers of loss of human contact.

Freedom of action and risk

"For fear of risk, too many people with dementia have a poorer quality of life." *Barbara Pointon, consultation respondent*

"My mother insisted for a long time that she could cook for herself … having seen some burnt pans my instinct was to switch off the cooker at the mains and 'pretend' it was broken, but she delighted in being able to accomplish something for herself. An independent assessment confirmed that her sense of achievement outweighed the risks involved, with smoke detectors etc in place to try to ensure her safety as best we could." *Alzheimer's Society (quoting one of its members), consultation respondent*

"Anybody looking after someone with dementia would naturally make sure they are never put at risk." *Anonymous consultation respondent*

"The participants' first instinct in balancing protection of basic freedom and protection from harm was to find the middle ground: an action that would preserve at least the appearance or feeling of freedom whilst allowing family members to assure themselves of the person's safety." *Opinion Leader, summarising the approach taken by participants in the Nuffield Council on Bioethics' Deliberative Workshop on dementia, August 2008*

6.13 Taking risks is an inherent part of our everyday lives, and a life without any form of risk is unimaginable. Those caring for people with dementia however, may often feel the need to do all they can to reduce risk to an absolute minimum. This may be because of a natural tendency to be more protective of others than one is of oneself.[328] It may also, in the context of care homes and other residential services, be linked with concerns about repercussions, including legal repercussions, if a person suffers harm that might have been averted.[329] Unfortunately, minimising risk often means forgoing benefits and restricting freedom, which in turn may be highly detrimental both to the person's sense of autonomy and to their overall well-being.

6.14 It was clear from our consultation responses that the issue of how best to balance freedom and protection for a person with dementia causes much anxiety among carers. Research by the American Alzheimer's Association showed that this issue is also important to people with early-stage dementia. In particular, much anger was expressed by research participants about attempts to control their behaviour and minimise risk in a way which they saw as both excessive and demeaning.[330] In later stages of dementia, it is sometimes argued that 'difficult' or 'unusual'

---

[328] See, for example, evidence about research involvement where proxies tend to be more protective than the person would have been themselves, including Muncie HL Jr, Magaziner J, Hebel JR and Warren JW (1997) Proxies' decisions about clinical research participation for their charges *Journal of the American Geriatric Association* **45**: 929–33.

[329] See, for example, the discussion of the 'duty of care' owed to people living in residential care in Commission for Social Care Inspection (2007) *Rights, Risks and Restraints: An exploration into the use of restraint in the care of older people* (London: Commission for Social Care Inspection), at p50, where it is emphasised that a 'duty of care' does *not* mean keeping people safe from every possible risk.

[330] Alzheimer's Association (2008) *Voices of Alzheimer's Disease* (Chicago: Alzheimer's Association), p17.

behaviours on the part of the person with dementia are often a response to what is perceived as over-controlling and restrictive behaviour on the part of the carer.[331]

6.15 Dilemmas relating to risk taking and freedom of action arise throughout dementia, from when early symptoms first appear to much later stages. The question of whether a person with early dementia should continue driving, for example, can be highly problematic. This involves balancing likely risks to both self and others with the freedom of the person with dementia.[332] The Alzheimer's Association research identified how very differently individuals respond to what many experience as a major blow to their independence: some give up driving almost immediately, while others continue as long as possible and strongly resist suggestions that they are not safe.[333] Later in dementia, the balance between facilitating a person's wishes and protecting their safety may arise in terms of safe walking outside,[334] or when considering how to meet a person's desire for privacy in the bathroom despite concern about the danger of falling. Similar concerns arise at all stages of dementia in terms of independent living.

6.16 These dilemmas arise in part because there may be conflicts between the autonomy interests of people with dementia, their own well-being interests, and the interests and safety of others. There may, furthermore, be conflicts even when considering only one interest. For example, although high levels of physical safety are an important aspect of well-being, the constraints, lack of privacy and lack of variety in life which may often accompany protective measures may significantly interfere with well-being. It may be valuable to recognise, too, that 'feeling safe' contributes to well-being.[335]

6.17 In recognising that a balance must be struck between enabling a person to live their life in the way they wish, promoting their well-being, protecting their safety, and protecting the safety and interests of others, we would like to emphasise the following points:

- Risks cannot be avoided completely. Some degree of risk is inevitable in everyday living.
- Encouraging independence and freedom of action is an important part of providing good quality of care and of supporting a person's autonomy. Restrictions that limit these freedoms may have an adverse effect both on the person's autonomy and on their general well-being, even where they are imposed with the aim of protecting the person.
- It is clearly important that those providing care for people with dementia assess and manage risk appropriately, and care providers are accordingly required to carry out 'risk assessments' for all those in their care.[336] However, the nature of a 'risk assessment' is such that it is very easy to focus only on the possible risks and how they can be minimised or eliminated, without considering what opportunities and benefits are being forgone as a result. For this reason we believe that 'risk assessment' is a misguided term and should be replaced by 'risk-benefit assessment'.

[331] See, for example, Stokes G (2007) *Challenging Behaviour in Dementia: A person-centred approach* (Brackley, UK: Speechmark Publishing Ltd.); the point was also made at the Working Party's fact-finding meeting with people on the front-line of dementia care, 10 July 2008.

[332] Drivers' Medical Group, Driver and Vehicle Licensing Agency (2009) *For Medical Practitioners: At a glance guide to the current medical standards of fitness to drive* (Swansea: Driver and Vehicle Licensing Agency); Alzheimer's Society (2008) *Driving and Dementia*, Factsheet 439 (London: Alzheimer's Society), available at: http://alzheimers.org.uk/factsheet/439.

[333] Alzheimer's Association (2008) *Voices of Alzheimer's Disease* (Chicago: Alzheimer's Association), p16.

[334] Robinson L, Hutchings D, Corner L *et al.* (2007) Balancing rights and risks: conflicting perspectives in the management of wandering in dementia *Health, Risk & Society* **9(4)**: 389–406.

[335] Qureshi H and Henwood M (2000) *Older People's Definitions of Quality Services* (York: Joseph Rowntree Foundation), available at: www.jrf.org.uk/sites/files/jrf/185935338x.pdf.

[336] The Regulation and Quality Improvement Authority (2008) *Residential Care Homes: Minimum standards* (Belfast: Department of Health, Social Services and Public Safety), standard 3.4; The Scottish Government (2007) *National Care Standards: Care homes for older people* (Edinburgh: The Scottish Government), standards 3, 4, and 9; Welsh Assembly Government (2004) *National Minimum Standards for Care Homes for Older People* (Cardiff: Welsh Assembly Government), standard 6.3; Department of Health (2003) *Care Homes for Older People: National minimum standards – care homes regulations* (London: The Stationery Office), standard 3.3.

■ A 'risk-benefit assessment' considers both the possible risks and the potential benefits of a proposed activity, service or facility. The one can then be weighed against the other, enabling some risk to be accepted in order to achieve a particular benefit.

■ Such an approach encourages those providing care to consider what is best for *this* particular person (taking into account others' safety and interests where appropriate), rather than simply choosing the course of action which, in the abstract, appears to pose the lowest level of risk. It also discourages an approach to risk which is based more on the convenience of others than on the needs of the person with dementia. A risk-benefit assessment further encourages the person carrying it out to consider the risks of *not* providing or permitting the activity in question: for example the risks of walking outside or alone should be weighed against the risks of prolonged sitting, boredom and frustration.

■ The importance of considering risks and benefits together is also relevant when considering the well-being of a group of people. Facilities such as kitchenette areas in care home lounges, encouraging more independence and a more home-like feel, or ornamental pools in care home gardens, may have a significant part to play in the quality of life of people living in the home, and such benefits must be taken properly into account when assessing and managing any risks they might also pose.

Recommendation 10: We recommend that the UK Departments of Health and the four bodies regulating adult social care in the UK[337] should require care providers to consider risks not in isolation but in the context of a risk-benefit assessment. Such risk-benefit assessments should explicitly take into account the well-being and autonomy of the person with dementia, as well as their need for protection from physical harm and the needs and interests of others. The term 'risk assessment' should be replaced by 'risk-benefit assessment' in order to highlight the importance of benefits which may be lost in the attempt to reduce risk.

6.18 We recognise that those providing paid care in either residential or home settings are potentially subject to criticism, and even legal action, if a person with dementia suffers harm as a result of a particular decision taken to promote their independence or freedom of action. These concerns might understandably lead to cautious decisions being taken that err on the side of excessive restriction of freedom in the name of safety. We suggest that a focus on *benefits*, as well as risks, as discussed above, together with good communication between professionals, care workers and families, should help in making decisions which best support the person with dementia to have a good quality of life. Such discussions should, wherever possible, include the person with dementia themselves.

Sexual relationships and sexual disinhibition

"Healthcare services need to take on board that people still have sex over the age of retirement and build this into assessment and care needs for people, including the privacy and intimate space to have mutually consenting sexual relationships." *United Kingdom Psychiatric Pharmacy Group and The College of Mental Health Pharmacists, consultation respondents*

"Should I allow this person with dementia privately to have a [new] sexual relationship, or should I tell the family to allow them to decide to forbid it?" *Professor June Andrews, Director, The Dementia Services Development Centre, University of Stirling, consultation respondent*

---

[337] The Care Quality Commission in England; the Care and Social Services Inspectorate Wales; the Care Commission in Scotland; and the Regulation and Quality Improvement Authority in Northern Ireland.

6.19 Intimate sexual relationships often continue into old age, with research showing that many men and women remain sexually active well into their eighties.[338] Little, however, is yet known about how couples where one or both partners have dementia make adjustments to accommodate their sexual relationship as the dementia progresses, or about the effects of specific types of dementia on the ability to engage in a sexual relationship. Respect for both a person's autonomy and their well-being demands that such relationships should be respected. Neither carers nor care workers should make the assumption that the sexual aspect of a long-standing relationship between a person with dementia and their partner is no longer important or consensual, and care homes in particular should take steps to ensure that their residents have the privacy to continue such relationships to the extent that they wish. While the rational ability of a person to consent to sexual activity is likely to decline as dementia progresses, it would be quite inappropriate for professionals to intervene in a relationship of a long-standing consensual nature, unless there are genuine concerns as to the willingness of one partner to participate.[339]

6.20 Difficulties can arise, however, where the relationship in question is new, or relatively new. These may include concerns about the consensual nature of the relationship and the difficulties that some members of the individual's family may face in dealing with the fact that their relative has a desire to form a new relationship in a care home context.[340] Depending on the degree of cognitive impairment on either side, such relationships may reflect genuine attraction between two individuals (including where a spouse is still alive); they may be based on mistaken beliefs on one or both sides (for example that the other person is in fact their spouse); or they may potentially be abusive. In some circumstances, however, what looks like a 'sexual relationship' may in fact simply be the result of disorientation: a person with dementia may simply have gone into the wrong bedroom and unwittingly got into bed with the occupant.

6.21 Deciding if, when, and how to intervene in a new sexual relationship may be very difficult, and a case conference involving relevant care workers and professionals may be a useful way of coming to a decision. If it is clear that the relationship is unwanted, or harmful, for one of the people involved, then that person should be appropriately protected. If this is not the case, then, while it will often be appropriate to involve family members who know the person well, their distaste for the idea of a new relationship starting late in life should not be sufficient reason for intervening. Any decision must be made on the basis of the person's own autonomy and well-being, bearing in mind that the person's own past views about sexual fidelity will be an important part of assessing their autonomy interests.

6.22 It is also crucial for those providing care to be aware that some people with dementia (7% in one survey[341] but less than 2% in another[342]) may behave in a way that is seen as sexually 'inappropriate' or ambiguous, for example through exposing themselves in public, making sexually explicit comments, or inappropriate touching. Such behaviour may result from the damage to parts of the brain which control and inhibit behaviour which would normally be kept private (see paragraph 1.8), or may simply be linked with the person's disorientation in time or space: for example a person may expose themselves in public because they need to go to the toilet and not for any

---

[338] Tessler Lindau S, Schumm LP, Laumann EO et al. (2007) A study of sexuality and health in older adults in the United States New England Journal of Medicine **357**: 762–74.

[339] For a more detailed discussion of this issue, see Bouman WP (2008) Sexuality in later life, in Oxford Textbook of Old Age Psychiatry, Jacoby R, Oppenheimer C, Dening T and Thomas A (Editors) (Oxford: Oxford University Press), pp689–707.

[340] Ehrenfeld M, Bronner G, Tabak N et al. (1999) Sexuality among institutionalised elderly patients with dementia Nursing Ethics **6(2)**: 144–9.

[341] Burns A, Jacoby R and Levy R (1990) Psychiatric phenomena in Alzheimer's disease IV: disorders of behaviour British Journal of Psychiatry **157**: 86–94.

[342] Alagiakrishnan K, Lim D, Brahim A et al. (2005) Sexually inappropriate behaviour in demented elderly people Postgraduate Medical Journal **81**: 463–6.

sexual motivation.[343] It has been noted that there will often be a fine line between 'appropriate' and 'inappropriate' behaviour, depending on the values and concerns of those working in the care home and family members, and that it is important to avoid stereotypical assumptions of older adults as asexual.[344] It is also clearly inappropriate to label behaviour as 'sexual' when in fact it arises out of discomfort, disorientation or toileting difficulties. Where behaviour is genuinely sexually inappropriate, professionals and care workers should feel confident in managing it in a consistent way, while seeking to treat the person concerned with respect.[345]

Truth telling

"I felt fully justified in telling lies if it prevented my mother going through even more distress." *Mrs Linda Tolson, consultation respondent*

"I don't think it helps anyone to lie about anything." *Anonymous consultation respondent*

"There comes a point when conversation is more important than cold truth and a conversation about a person is more constructive than living through bereavement day after day." *Older People and Disability Team, Social Care and Learning Department, Bracknell Forest Council, consultation respondent*

"[A] sensible balance of truth and 'white lies.'" *Anonymous consultation respondent*

6.23 As the quotes above suggest, responses to the consultation question on the subject of truth telling ranged from an absolute prohibition on telling lies, to viewing well-being as paramount. Other responses portrayed the anguish relatives of people with dementia experience in trying to do the 'right thing', and highlighted that, in many cases, the difference between 'the truth' and a 'white lie' may not be as clear as first appears.

6.24 The ethical reasoning behind most responses was based on concern for the well-being of the person with dementia, with conflicts experienced between the desire to maintain trust (especially in the context of long-standing relationships built on trust) and avoiding distress. These considerations of the interests of the person with dementia run alongside both beliefs about the moral importance of telling the truth and practical concerns about how to get through the day.

6.25 The issue of truth telling highlights the difficulties inherent in determining what course of action is genuinely in a person's best interests, both in the immediate and longer term. Avoiding distress is clearly important for the person's day-to-day happiness, while many will feel strongly that 'not being lied to' is an important aspect of the more objective elements of a person's well-being and autonomy interests. Questions of trust are particularly difficult. Some argue that failing to tell the truth is a breach of trust and serves to undermine the remaining grip the person with dementia may have on the everyday world.[346] Others point out that telling the straightforward truth in circumstances where the person with dementia will not believe it may equally undermine trust because the person will think that they are being lied to.[347] For care workers and professionals there is the added issue of whether telling lies undermines the integrity of professional care,[348] and

[343] See, for example, Stokes G (2007) *Challenging Behaviour in Dementia: A person-centred approach* (Brackley, UK: Speechmark Publishing Ltd), at p17 and p113.
[344] Bouman WP (2008) Sexuality in later life, in *Oxford Textbook of Old Age Psychiatry*, Jacoby R, Oppenheimer C, Dening T and Thomas A (Editors) (Oxford: Oxford University Press), pp689–707, at 701.
[345] See, for example, Ballard C, O'Brien J, James I and Swann A (Editors) (2001) *Dementia: Management of behavioural and psychological symptoms* (Oxford: Oxford University Press), p279.
[346] Schermer M (2007) Nothing but the truth? On truth and deception in dementia care *Bioethics* **21(1)**: 13–22.
[347] Working Party's fact-finding meeting with Professor Dawn Brooker from the Bradford Dementia Group, 30 Sept 2008.
[348] Schermer M (2007) Nothing but the truth? On truth and deception in dementia care *Bioethics* **21(1)**: 13–22.

for all concerned in providing care, paid or unpaid, there is the concern that failing to tell the truth is detrimental to their own moral well-being.

6.26 As we made clear at the beginning of this Chapter, we do not believe that there is a single answer to this dilemma. Telling the truth is clearly an important moral value, and telling the truth will always be the natural starting point. However, in circumstances where significant distress or anger is caused by verbally truthful answers to questions, because of the person's cognitive problems, then it may be more humane to find responses that evade or offer only a partial answer to the person's question, in order to minimise distress. Only very rarely would a direct lie be the best or only option.

6.27 In many cases it may also be appropriate to seek to respond to the *emotions* involved, even if this involves some degree of latitude with the factual truth. Indeed, it could be argued that such an approach is truthful, in that it responds to the *actual* concerns of the person with dementia, regardless of the language in which it is clothed. One carer, for example, described to us how he would always tell his wife that he was 'going shopping' at the end of a visit to her care home, because she understood that to mean that he was going but would be back sometime soon. Saying a simple 'goodbye', on the other hand, caused significant distress, presumably because it was interpreted as indicating a much longer separation than would in fact be the case.[349]

Restraint

"I remember the University of – somewhere – hospital, I got so agitated that they had to strap me down … I did hate that … I remember that night as one of the very worst nights in all the time I've lived." [350]

"My father was moved without warning from one acute ward to another, and he naturally became distressed, and complained loudly. The reaction of the nurses was to surround him with furniture, and get security staff to stand over him." *Anonymous consultation respondent*

"… sometimes it is essential. What else would you do if a patient was assaulting another patient?" *Anonymous consultation respondent*

6.28 The issue of restraint often arises in the context of dementia, either because restraint is seen as a possible way of protecting the person with dementia (for example with the aim of preventing them from falling) or because of concerns about the safety of others (for example where the person with dementia is perceived to be acting in a threatening way). In some circumstances, the person with dementia may have the capacity to understand why a particular restraint is being suggested for their own safety and may consent to its use. Such uses of restraint are usually unproblematic. However, in many cases the person with dementia may not be in a position to consent, or restraint may be used in order to control behaviour that others find difficult or alarming, and in such cases restraint may be experienced as highly demeaning and distressing. Yet, at times, those caring for a person with dementia may see no alternative but to use restraint.

Uses of restraint

6.29 The most obvious form of restraint is *physical restraint*. This may involve force, for example to control someone who is behaving aggressively; alternatively it may include equipment such as straps or lap belts. Less overt forms of restraint include placing a person in a chair which is too low

---

349 Bruce Bovill, responding to the Working Party's consultation.
350 Henderson CS (1998) *Partial View: An Alzheimer's journal* (Dallas: Southern Methodist University Press), p88.

for them to get out of without help, or locking doors to prevent people from leaving a room or building.[351] There may be significant physical and emotional risks of being physically restrained, coupled with a risk that restraint will become a vicious circle, with the distress and reaction to restraint putting a person at a greater risk of being repeatedly physically restrained in the future.[352] There is also the risk that physical restraint imposed with the aim of avoiding minor accidents may in fact lead to more serious outcomes, such as more serious accidents if a person tries to move despite the restraint mechanism, reduced mobility, pressure sores and depression.[353]

6.30 A number of pharmacological treatments, including anti-depressants, anti-anxiety medicines, mood-stabilising medicines and anti-psychotics may be used to calm and control the behaviour of a person with dementia by reducing their levels of activity or consciousness. Where these medicines are used primarily with the aim of controlling behaviour, rather than responding to symptoms such as anxiety or depression, this is sometimes known as *chemical restraint*.

6.31 Much has recently been written about the way the anti-psychotic drugs, in particular, have been overused in people with dementia,[354] and this is of particular concern given evidence that use of anti-psychotic medicines in people with Alzheimer's disease and dementia with Lewy bodies is associated with a shortened life expectancy.[355] The NICE/SCIE guidelines make clear that medication should be considered for 'behaviour that challenges' in the first instance only if there is severe distress or immediate risk of harm, with non-pharmacological approaches preferred in all other circumstances (see Box 1.2). However, it is important to keep a clear distinction between when these medicines are being used in response to particular symptoms, and when they are being used in the very short term as a form of restraint, as an alternative to physical restraint. In the first case, their use should be governed by the best practice guidance issued by NICE/SCIE and SIGN, while in the latter case they will additionally be governed by the law on restraint outlined below.

The law on restraint

"In drawing attention to the issue the law raises awareness of the undesirability of restraint but it provides little guidance as to the level and nature of appropriate restraint or circumstances in which it might be used." *Dr Hazel McHaffie, consultation respondent*

6.32 In England and Wales, the Mental Capacity Act governs cases where a person who lacks capacity is restrained by others. It allows restraint to be used only when it is necessary to prevent harm to the person lacking capacity and where it is a "proportionate" response to the likelihood of the person suffering harm, and to the seriousness of that harm.[356] The Act uses a wide definition of 'restraint': "the use or threat of force to help do an act which the person resists, or the restriction of the person's liberty of movement, whether or not they resist."[357] An authoritative commentary

---

[351] Depending on the circumstances (for example the time-scale involved, and the degree of control exerted over the person concerned), locking people in a room or building may in fact constitute 'deprivation of liberty', rather than restraint, and will be subject to additional safeguards.

[352] Wang W and Moyle W (2005) Physical restraint use on people with dementia: a review of the literature *Australian Journal of Advanced Nursing* **22(4)**: 46–52.

[353] Commission for Social Care Inspection (2007) *Rights, Risks and Restraints: An exploration into the use of restraint in the care of older people* (London: Commission for Social Care Inspection), p51.

[354] See, for example, All Party Parliamentary Group on Dementia (2008) *Always a Last Resort: Inquiry into the prescription of anti-psychotic drugs to people with dementia living in care homes* (London: Alzheimer's Society); Alldred DP, Petty DR, Bowie P, Zermansky AG and Raynor DK (2007) Antipsychotic prescribing patterns in care homes and relationship with dementia *Psychiatric Bulletin* **31(9)**: 329–32; Fossey J, Ballard C, Juszczak E *et al.* (2006) Effect of enhanced psychosocial care on antipsychotic use in nursing home residents with severe dementia: cluster randomised trial *British Medical Journal* **332**: 756–61.

[355] Ballard C, Hanney ML, Theodoulou M *et al.* (2009) The dementia antipsychotic withdrawal trial (DART-AD): long-term follow-up of a randomised placebo-controlled trial *Lancet Neurology* **8(2)**: 151–7; McKeith I, Fairbairn A, Perry R, Thompson P and Perry E (1992) Neuroleptic sensitivity in patients with senile dementia of Lewy body type *British Medical Journal* **305**: 673–8.

[356] ss6(2) and 6(3) Mental Capacity Act 2005, emphasised further in the Mental Capacity Act 2005 Code of Practice, chapter 6.41.

[357] s6(4) of the Mental Capacity Act, as summarised in the Mental Capacity Act 2005 Code of Practice, p290.

on the Act suggests that this may include many forms of restraint, both verbal and physical, "from shouting at someone, to holding them down to locking them in a room" and may also include "the prescribing of a sedative or other chemical restraint which restricts liberty of movement."[358] The Act clearly prohibits those providing care from restraining people with dementia simply in order to make their own tasks easier: there must be an objective reason for the restraint in order to prevent harm to the person with dementia. Moreover, the restraint must be "proportionate", that is, the need for the restraint must be sufficiently serious to justify such a serious response, and if less intrusive ways of dealing with the situation can be found, these should be preferred.

6.33 The Adults with Incapacity (Scotland) Act is silent on the issue of restraint in general, but states that "force and detention" may be used in connection with medical treatment only where it is immediately necessary.[359] As in England, the common law permits restraint if this is necessary to prevent immediate harm or in self-defence.[360] In all four countries of the UK, the regulations governing care homes forbid restraint unless it is "the only practicable means of securing the welfare of that or any other service user and there are exceptional circumstances."[361] Detailed guidance issued by the Mental Welfare Commission for Scotland makes clear that in Scotland this requirement should be interpreted as meaning that restraint should only ever be a "last resort, where there is absolutely no alternative."[362] The Northern Ireland consultation document setting out broad proposals for a new Mental Capacity Act states that the new legislation will make clear that "restraint will only be permitted if the person using it reasonably believes it is necessary to prevent harm and it is proportionate to the likelihood and seriousness of the harm."[363]

6.34 While the various Regulations governing the use of restraint in care homes in England, Wales, Scotland and Northern Ireland all limit the use of restraint to "exceptional" circumstances, where there is no alternative course of action, there is considerable anecdotal evidence that, in fact, restraint is much more widely used than this. An 'exploration' of restraint in English care homes, carried out in 2007 by the Commission for Social Care Inspection (CSCI), described many examples of restraint which appeared to be routine rather than exceptional, and the Commission cited "widespread suspicion" that restraint was often used not to ensure residents' safety but in order to help staff manage their workload.[364] Thus, although the Regulations are clear as to the exceptional nature of restraint, it is less clear that they are being respected in practice.

6.35 CSCI concluded its report with a set of principles which good restraint policies in care homes should include, emphasising that restraint should always "be the least restrictive option and undertaken for the shortest viable length of time", and recommended that its successor body (the Care Quality Commission) should continue to keep the issue of restraint under review. The guidance published by the Mental Welfare Commission in Scotland, on the other hand, is much more detailed, setting out

---

[358] Ashton G, Letts P, Oates L and Terrell M (2006) *Mental Capacity: The new law* (Bristol: Jordans), paragraph 2.133.

[359] s47(7)(a) Adults With Incapacity (Scotland) Act 2000.

[360] A summary of the common law is given in Mental Welfare Commission for Scotland (2006) *Rights, Risks and Limits to Freedom: Principles and good practice guidance for practitioners using restraint in residential care settings* (Edinburgh: Mental Welfare Commission for Scotland), Appendix 1.

[361] Regulation 13(7)(a) of the Care Homes Regulations 2001, SI 2001/3965, as amended; Regulation 4(1)(c) of the Regulation of Care (Requirements as to Care Services) (Scotland) Regulations 2002, SSI 2002/114, as amended; Regulation 14(5) of the Residential Care Homes Regulations (Northern Ireland) 2005, SR2005/161, as amended; Regulation 13(7) of the Care Homes (Wales) Regulations 2002, SI 2002/324(W.37), as amended.

[362] Mental Welfare Commission for Scotland (2006) *Rights, Risks and Limits to Freedom: Principles and good practice guidance for practitioners using restraint in residential care settings* (Edinburgh: Mental Welfare Commission for Scotland), p2.

[363] Northern Ireland Department of Health, Social Services and Public Safety (2009) *Legislative Framework for Mental Capacity and Mental Health Legislation in Northern Ireland: A policy consultation document* (Belfast: Northern Ireland Department of Health, Social Services and Public Safety), paragraph 5.1.

[364] Commission for Social Care Inspection (2007) *Rights, Risks and Restraints: An exploration into the use of restraint in the care of older people* (London: CSCI), pp39–40.

practical requirements which encourage the use of restraint only as a genuine exception to the norm. One example is the requirement that members of staff must be "in direct visual and verbal contact with the resident" during any time in which their movements are subject to restraint, thus automatically preventing the use of restraint as a way of dealing with staff shortages or pressures.[365]

Our approach

6.36 The issue of restraint, and when it is right to use it, will usually involve the balancing of several values (see paragraph 6.2). Clearly there have to be very good reasons to justify the use of restraint, and by specifically restricting the use of restraint to circumstances where it is "proportionate", the Mental Capacity Act highlights this point, as does the detailed guidance issued by the Mental Welfare Commission for Scotland. The regulations governing care homes throughout the United Kingdom arguably go further by emphasising the exceptional nature of restraint, although, as we note above, there is some evidence that these requirements are not reliably followed.

6.37 We note, however, that it is far from clear in many circumstances how the 'proportionality' principle in the Mental Capacity Act would work in practice, and that this lack of clarity poses real difficulties for those providing care, particularly carers, on a regular basis. For example, is it proportionate for a wife who cares alone for her husband with dementia to lock him in the house or in the car while she goes shopping, because she is not able to obtain any support to look after him in her absence and he might be at risk if he went out alone? Is it proportionate for her to leave him in a low chair which he cannot leave without help, in order to cook a meal in peace? Sometimes the real issue at stake is the availability of support for carers: what is needed is not reassurance about the proportionality of the form of restraint, but rather a sitting service for a few hours a week and some assistance in identifying activities which will occupy the person with dementia without the need for restraint. In many cases, however, such support will simply not be available, and there will always be less predictable circumstances or emergencies where a planned solution is unlikely to be applicable.

6.38 We have emphasised, throughout this Report, the equal value of people with dementia, the importance of promoting their autonomy and well-being, and the moral importance of demonstrating solidarity both with people who have dementia and with the family and friends who support them. We recognise that restraint is an immensely difficult and emotional issue that is often experienced as deeply degrading and de-humanising, and yet there may be times when carers feel they must use restraint. We suggest our focus on solidarity provides strong justification for the argument that support for carers that obviates the need for restraint should be regarded as a very high priority by local health and social services. While the Mental Capacity Act Code of Practice contains some useful advice about when the use of restraint is "proportionate", we also suggest that more explicit guidance, covering a much wider range of situations in the context of the home, would be very helpful.

Recommendation 11: We recommend that the Office of the Public Guardian, in association with the Department of Health, provide additional guidance to carers on when restraint might be considered to be "proportionate", either within the Mental Capacity Act Code of Practice or in the form of stand-alone guidance.

Recommendation 12: We recommend that the Commissions responsible for regulating social care within the United Kingdom ensure that detailed and practical guidance on the appropriate use of restraint in care homes, such as that produced by the Mental Welfare Commission for Scotland, is made readily available to all those working in this sector.

---

[365] Mental Welfare Commission for Scotland (2006) *Rights, Risks and Limits to Freedom: Principles and good practice guidance for practitioners using restraint in residential care settings* (Edinburgh: Mental Welfare Commission for Scotland), paragraph 3.1.19.

Recommendation 13: We further recommend that the UK Health Departments should draw specific attention to the importance of providing support to carers that will minimise the need for restraint in the domestic context, for example through guidance to health and social services organisations on needs assessment.[366]

Abuse by family or friends

"Should I respond to an apparent abuse of the patient by the carer, or do I remain silent, as the alternative institution is probably unpleasant and not what the patient would have wanted?" Professor June Andrews, Director, Dementia Services Development Centre, University of Stirling, consultation respondent

"[There is a] difficulty of establishing whether or not abuse has taken place, in the person's own home or in a care home." Guideposts Trust, consultation respondent

6.39 It is only relatively recently that the abuse of older people, both by their carers and by professionals or care workers, has been recognised as a serious issue.[367] It has since been shown that cognitive impairment is itself a significant risk factor for abuse,[368] and hence older people with dementia may be particularly vulnerable. The abuse of people with dementia by the family or friends involved in caring for them raises particular ethical issues, because of the complex relationships and dependencies involved, and this section will focus specifically on this aspect of abuse.

6.40 A clear picture of the scale either of elder abuse in general, or of the abuse of people with dementia in particular, remains elusive, in part because of varying definitions of elder abuse. In 2002, in its Toronto Declaration on the Global Prevention of Elder Abuse, the World Health Organization (WHO) adopted the definition used by the UK organisation Action on Elder Abuse: "a single or repeated act or lack of appropriate action occurring within any relationship where there is an expectation of trust, which causes harm or distress to an older person", and noted that it can be of various forms: "physical, psychological/emotional, sexual, financial or simply reflect intentional or unintentional neglect."[369] By contrast, other definitions emphasise the intent of the person perpetrating the abuse, or limit the definition to 'harm or a serious risk of harm', rather than the wider 'harm or distress.'[370] An overview published in 2008 of empirical studies of 'maltreatment' of people with dementia by carers, covering factors such as emotional or verbal abuse, financial exploitation, and various forms of neglect and violence, cited figures of physical abuse of the person with dementia of between five per cent and 12 per cent (47% where the research was carried out among those being referred for respite care) and emotional abuse of between 11 per cent and 52 per cent.[371]

---

[366] See, for example, the guidance issued by the Department of Health in England on the 'single assessment process', available at: www.dh.gov.uk/en/SocialCare/Chargingandassessment/SingleAssessmentProcess/DH_079509.

[367] See, for example, Baker AA (1975) Granny battering *Modern Geriatrics* **8**: 20–4 and Burston GR (1975) Granny battering *British Medical Journal* **3**: 592, both cited in Cooney C and Wrigley M (1996) Abuse of the elderly with dementia *Irish Journal of Psychological Medicine* **13(3)**: 94–6.

[368] Cooney C and Wrigley M (1996) Abuse of the elderly with dementia *Irish Journal of Psychological Medicine* **13(3)**: 94–6; Hirsch RD and Vollhardt BR (2008) Elder maltreatment, in *Oxford Textbook of Old Age Psychiatry*, Jacoby R, Oppenheimer C, Dening T and Thomas A (Editors), pp731–45 at 735.

[369] World Health Organization (2002) The *Toronto Declaration on the Global Prevention of Elder Abuse* (Geneva: World Health Organization); also see Action on Elder Abuse (2008) *What is Elder Abuse?* (London: Action on Elder Abuse), available at: www.elderabuse.org.uk/Useful%20downloads/leaflets/whatisleaflet.pdf.

[370] See, for example, the definition used by the National Center on Elder Abuse: "any knowing, intentional, or negligent act by a caregiver or any other person that causes harm or a serious risk of harm to a vulnerable adult", available at: www.ncea.aoa.gov/NCEAroot/Main_Site/FAQ/Questions.aspx.

[371] Hirsch RD and Vollhardt BR (2008) Elder maltreatment, in *Oxford Textbook of Old Age Psychiatry*, Jacoby R, Oppenheimer C, Dening T and Thomas A (Editors) (Oxford: Oxford University Press), pp731–45, table 39.3.

6.41 The WHO definition of elder abuse is valuable in that it highlights the wide range of contexts in which harm may occur to older people. It should, however, be emphasised that since this definition has been interpreted as including behaviours such as using a harsh tone or insulting the person with dementia, or threatening to send them to a care home, the figures on abuse must also be interpreted in this light. For example, a 2009 survey of abuse of people with dementia by carers, using the WHO definition of 'abuse', was widely reported as showing that over half the carers of people with dementia were guilty of abuse.[372] In the detailed breakdown of forms of abuse included in the study, however, the percentage of carers who admitted physical abuse was one per cent of those participating in the study, with a further three per cent saying that they had been afraid they might hit or hurt the person for whom they were caring, but had not done so. Thirty-three per cent of carers, on the other hand, reported behaviours that the authors categorised as 'psychological' abuse at least sometimes in the previous three months: these behaviours including screaming or swearing at the person for whom they cared, and threatening to stop caring for them or send them to a care home.

6.42 It is clearly very important to make the point that abuse can take many different forms, and that repeated verbal abuse and threats may be as harmful and distressing as physical violence. Moreover, studies such as the 2009 research cited above may underestimate serious cases of physical abuse, or malicious forms of abuse, which people are reluctant to acknowledge. Nevertheless, this study does suggest that headline figures about the prevalence of abuse in dementia should be treated with caution. The nature of the distress, the intent of those causing the distress, and the background circumstances will all be important factors in determining how best to combat the abuse. Moreover, while physical violence will always be a source of immediate concern, it is important to note that the distress caused by what is described as 'psychological' abuse will vary enormously: in some households a husband and wife may always have shouted at each other, and may continue to do so without harm, while in others the person with dementia may experience significant distress from raised or angry voices.

6.43 The Alzheimer's Society has noted that, in many cases, behaviour which is distressing or harmful to the person with dementia may be unintentional, perhaps due to a lack of understanding about dementia and its impact, and not because the carers of the person with dementia are cruel or malicious.[373] In other cases the harm or distress may result from excessive stress on carers, owing to exhaustion, ill-health and lack of support, especially where behaviour on the part of the person with dementia may sometimes be deeply frustrating, threatening,[374] or indeed violent.[375] In some cases, these problems will be exacerbated by an already poor relationship between the person with dementia and a family member who has felt coerced into taking on the role of carer. The need to intervene in order to protect the person with dementia remains the same, regardless of the intent of the person causing the harm; however, the action necessary to protect the person may be quite different.

6.44 When professionals suspect that a person with dementia is suffering harm from a carer or other family member or friend, they have both a legal and an ethical duty to act to protect the person

---

[372] Cooper C, Selwood A, Blanchard M *et al.* (2009) Abuse of people with dementia by family carers: representative cross sectional study *British Medical Journal* **338**: b155; Daily Express (23 Jan 2009) *Dementia sufferers abused – survey*, available at: www.express. co.uk/posts/view/81349; The Guardian (23 Jan 2009) *Over 50% of carers admit to elder abuse*, available at: www.guardian.co.uk/ society/2009/jan/23/elder-abuse-dementia.

[373] Alzheimer's Society (2008) *Uncovering Abuse in the Dementia Care Environment* (London: Alzheimer's Society).

[374] See, for example, the YouGov survey carried out in December 2008 where 17 per cent of carers said they 'sometimes' felt threatened by the person for whom they were caring and two per cent said they 'often' felt threatened: YouGov (2009) *Alzheimer's – You Gov/ Channel 4 survey results* (London: YouGov/Channel 4), available at: www.yougov.co.uk/extranets/ygarchives/content/pdf/C4%20 results%20alzheimers.pdf.

[375] Hirsch RD and Vollhardt BR (2008) Elder maltreatment, in *Oxford Textbook of Old Age Psychiatry*, Jacoby R, Oppenheimer C, Dening T and Thomas A (Editors) (Oxford: Oxford University Press), pp731–45, table 39.3.

with dementia as a 'vulnerable adult'.[376] While a careful assessment may sometimes lead to the conclusion that the only way to protect the person's interests is by removing them from their current home, this outcome should never be assumed in advance. The autonomy and well-being interests of the person with dementia may be highly complex, and any benefits associated from a long-standing relationship must be weighed in the balance along with the nature and extent of the harm. Where it seems clear that the person with dementia does obtain benefit from their relationship with the person involved, then the focus should be on supporting the family or household as a whole with the aim of improving their knowledge of dementia and easing their burden of care, which may be what led them to lose control. We suggest that our recommendation in Chapter 3 (see paragraph 3.12) that professionals should treat carers as 'partners in care' will be of much positive benefit in avoiding and minimising harmful behaviour, by ensuring that carers feel appropriately supported and able to ask for help *before* a crisis is reached.

6.45 While some abuse will undoubtedly be of a malicious and criminal nature, there is considerable evidence as to the role played by ignorance, stress, ill-health and exhaustion on the part of carers. Allegations or evidence of abuse must always be thoroughly investigated and action taken to protect the person with dementia. At the same time it must be recognised that abuse and neglect may be the result of unmanageable pressure on the carer. **Our focus on solidarity emphasises the need both to act to protect the person with dementia and to support their carer where the person with dementia continues to benefit from their care. We suggest that these concerns add further weight to the importance of providing appropriate information, advice and peer support services to all those caring for people with dementia, as highlighted in Chapters 3, 6 and 7 (see paragraphs 3.25–3.29, 6.3 and 7.18).**

---

[376] See, for example, the 'No Secrets' guidance in England: Department of Health and Home Office (2000) *No Secrets: Guidance on developing and implementing multi-agency policies and procedures to protect vulnerable adults from abuse* (London: Department of Health), available at: www.dh.gov.uk/en/Publicationsandstatistics/Publications/PublicationsPolicyAndGuidance/DH_4008486.

Chapter 7

The needs of carers

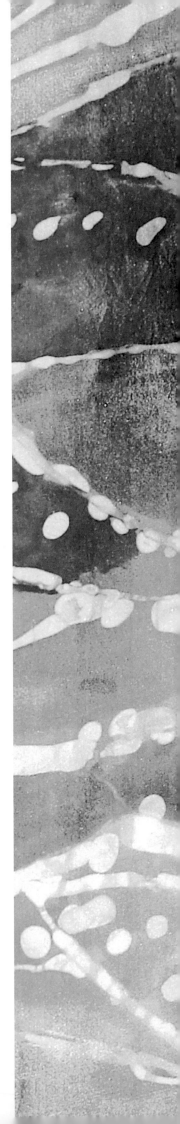

Chapter 7 – The needs of carers

"Although there is no standard definition of family caregiving, it is understood to involve providing extraordinary care, often outside the bounds of what is usual in family relationships."[377]

"… the informal family caregiver is a tribute to the human spirit. He or she is an altruist in the full sense of caring for another at considerable inconvenience to self."[378]

Introduction: the role of carers

7.1 A 'carer' is defined in the UK Government's Carer's Strategy as someone who "spends a significant proportion of their life providing unpaid support to family or … friends."[379] An analysis of carers in England derived from the 2001 census found that the majority of carers are of working age, although one in six are over 65, and that half live with the person for whom they provide care.[380]

7.2 For many people with dementia, the support they receive from carers will be their main source of assistance. The National Audit Office reports that there are some 476,000 unpaid carers in England supporting people with dementia,[381] and the 2007 *Dementia UK* report estimated that on average people with dementia receive 24 hours of care per week from carers, with that figure rising to 60 hours for those needing the most care.[382] A survey by Alzheimer Europe similarly reported that half of carers of people with late-stage dementia spend more than ten hours each day caring,[383] while over 80 per cent of the total care received by people with dementia in one Swedish study was provided by informal, rather than paid, carers.[384]

7.3 The support provided by a carer for a person with dementia will vary enormously depending on the nature and progress of the person's dementia, on the capabilities of the carer, and on what other assistance, if any, is available. It may include helping the person with some or all activities of daily living, from intimate personal care to housework; supporting the person in meaningful occupation; providing constant reassurance where the person fears being alone; helping with, or managing, financial and legal matters; and many other forms of support. Providing this level of constant support takes a great deal of time, hard work and compassion, and may often be emotionally and physically exhausting. A study of carers of people with dementia, stroke and Parkinson's disease found that the most frequently reported problems associated with caring were the disorganisation of household routines, difficulties with going away for holidays, restrictions on social life, and disturbances of sleep.[385]

7.4 In Chapter 2 we set out our ethical framework, highlighting our belief that a good quality of life is possible with dementia, but that in order to achieve this, significant support will be required

---

[377] Yap LKP, Seow CCD, Henderson LM and Goh YN (2005) Family caregivers and caregiving in dementia *Reviews in Clinical Gerontology* **15**: 263–71.

[378] Post S (2000) *Ethical Issues from Diagnosis to Dying: The moral challenge of Alzheimer's disease*, 2nd Edition (Baltimore: Johns Hopkins University Press), p25.

[379] HM Government (2008) *Carers at the Heart of 21st Century Families and Communities: "A caring system on your side. A life of your own"* (London: Department of Health), p19.

[380] Audit Commission (2004) *Support for Carers of Older People* (London: Audit Commission), p2.

[381] National Audit Office (2007) *Improving Services and Support for People with Dementia* (Norwich: The Stationery Office), p9.

[382] Knapp M and Prince M (King's College London and London School of Economics) (2007) *Dementia UK* (London: Alzheimer's Society), p66.

[383] Alzheimer Europe (2006) *Who Cares? The state of dementia care in Europe* (Luxembourg: Alzheimer Europe).

[384] Wimo A, von Strauss E, Nordberg G, Sassi F and Johansson L (2002) Time spent on informal and formal care giving for persons with dementia in Sweden *Health Policy* **61**: 255–68.

[385] Thommessen B, Aarsland D, Braekhus A *et al*. (2002) The psychosocial burden on spouses of the elderly with stroke, dementia and Parkinson's disease *International Journal of Geriatric Psychiatry* **17(1)**: 78–84.

to promote both the person's autonomy and their well-being. At the same time, we emphasised that the autonomy and well-being of carers were also morally important. Unlike care workers and professionals, a carer's responsibilities will often continue day and night and this may have very significant practical consequences: for example, additional stress and sheer exhaustion caused by broken nights may seriously affect both the health of the carer and their ability to provide care in the way that they would ideally like to do.[386] More fundamentally, however, it is crucial to recognise that the life of the person with dementia and their carer will often be very closely entwined, particularly where informal care is being provided by a partner, or by a relative living in the same house.

7.5   In such circumstances, the interests of the person being cared for and the person providing the care will often be inseparable, and this may have significant implications for how the various needs and interests at stake are balanced and compromises sought. Moreover, in providing care to a partner, close family member or friend, carers have to contend with their own complex emotions resulting, for example, from the changes in their relationship with the person with dementia, or from the loss of cherished future plans.[387]

7.6   While the pressure placed on carers by their caring role should not be underestimated, it is important also to highlight that for many carers the experience of caring for their relative or friend has many positive aspects.[388] Caring is often a key part of family relationships, and may offer carers an opportunity to express feelings of love, and also to act altruistically. Descriptions of caring recently published in the health care press by two individual carers, each of whom provided care to their wives with dementia, highlight some of these positive aspects:

"Caring does not constitute a cure, but it certainly can reveal one's inner strengths. It has its own rewards."[389]

"We [husband and wife] have been marked by a special kind of pain. But we have also experienced a deepening sense of responsibility, gratitude for all that we had lived through together, love, solidarity, and a shared sensibility that we have resisted what is beyond our control and are, individually and collectively, more for it."[390]

As the second quotation illustrates, 'caring' should not automatically be seen as a one-way process: for many people with dementia and their carers, the experience of being cared for and providing care will be closely tied up with the nature of their relationship. Indeed, as we note in Chapter 2 (see paragraph 2.45), the person with dementia should not be portrayed simply as a passive recipient of care, but rather as someone who has the potential to continue participating in family life, albeit in different ways from before.

Attitudes and beliefs about caring

"People find themselves looking after a confused person at home for many different reasons – out of love, from a sense of duty, perhaps because they feel they have no choice. Some find assuming responsibility relatively easy. Others come increasingly to resent it."[391]

[386] Dauvilliers Y (2007) Insomnia in patients with neurodegenerative conditions *Sleep Medicine* **8(4)**: S27–S34.

[387] See, for example, Schneider J, Murray J, Banerjee S and Mann A (1999) EUROCARE: a cross-national study of co-resident spouse carers for people with Alzheimer's disease: I – Factors associated with carer burden *International Journal of Geriatric Psychiatry* **14(8)**: 651–61.

[388] Netto NR, Goh JYN and Yap PLK (2009) Growing and gaining through caring for a loved one with dementia *Dementia* **8(2)**: 245–61.

[389] Lamont J (2008) Remembering the dance *Journal of Dementia Care* **16(2)**: 11.

[390] Kleinman A (2009) Caregiving: the odyssey of becoming more human *The Lancet* **373**: 292–3.

[391] Department of Health (2007) *Who Cares? Information and support for the carers of people with dementia* (London: Department of Health), p15.

"The reaction of the family and friends to the diagnosis can be crucial to the carer and patient. If it is good and positive, and accepted as an illness with no known cure as yet but one that will have its good and bad times, life for the carer and the patient can be very rewarding." *Jean Burnard, consultation respondent*

7.7 Most carers do not plan to be a carer, and nor do they receive special education about dementia or the effects it may have on their own lives. Indeed, a person will often not make a specific conscious decision to take on a caring role; rather it will evolve out of a relationship as a result of shifting levels of dependency.[392] Some people dislike being classified as 'carers' in the very early stages of dementia, seeing themselves as acting as caring partners, relatives or friends, rather than taking on a new role with a new name.[393]

7.8 Like the experience of dementia itself, the personal experience of being a carer, and the extent to which the positive aspects of providing care are outweighed by the physical and emotional burdens, is likely to be affected by a wide range of factors. These potentially include the personal characteristics of all involved, the nature of their relationships, the needs of the person with dementia, and the level of support received from others. In particular, the carer's beliefs about caring are likely to affect how the role is experienced.

7.9 One UK-based study in 2008 of three different ethnic groups classified attitudes to caring as 'traditional', where caring within the family was seen as natural, expected and virtuous, and 'non-traditional', where the carer perceived their own life as being 'on hold' while providing care and did not necessarily expect to derive reward or pleasure from caring. It found that while all carers in the study experienced health difficulties (particularly linked with exhaustion) as a result of their caring role, a more 'traditional' attitude helped carers find rewards in their relationship with the person for whom they were caring, and to feel that their lives, although changed, were ongoing. Although 'traditional' views were more common among carers of south Asian or Caribbean origin than among white British carers, 'traditional' and 'non-traditional' attitudes were identified among all three ethnic groups studied, thus emphasising the need for professionals to consider the specific needs and experiences of individual carers, without making prior assumptions about their likely attitude to caring.[394]

7.10 Where one person within a family or social circle takes on primary responsibility for providing care, the attitudes and assumptions about care within the wider family or network may also have a significant impact on the main carer. The extent to which the main carer feels supported may depend to a significant degree on how the rest of the family unit reacts both to the person with dementia and their carer. On the one hand, relatives outside the relationship between the main carer and the person with dementia may decide what the person with dementia and their main carer need, without first consulting them.[395] On the other hand, family members who have only limited contact with the person with dementia may underestimate how much support the person needs in day-to-day living, and hence fail to understand the degree of pressure under which the main carer is living.[396] Again, distinctions between 'traditional' and 'non-traditional' attitudes to

[392] Gillies B (2000) Acting up: role ambiguity and the legal recognition of carers *Ageing and Society* **20**: 429–44.

[393] Goldsteen M, Abma T, Oeseburg B *et al.* (2007) What is it to be a daughter? Identities under pressure in dementia care *Bioethics* **21(1)**: 1–12.

[394] Lawrence V, Murray J, Samsi K and Banerjee S (2008) Attitudes and support needs of Black Caribbean, south Asian and White British carers of people with dementia in the UK *British Journal of Psychiatry* **193**: 240–6.

[395] Zarit SH and Zarit JM (2008) Flexibility and change: the fundamentals for families coping with dementia, in *Excellence in Dementia Care: Research into practice*, Downs M and Bowers B (Editors) (Maidenhead, UK: Open University Press), p93.

[396] See, for example, NHS Health Scotland (2008) *Coping with Dementia: A practical handbook for carers* (Edinburgh and Glasgow: Health Scotland), p19.

the role of the family in providing care may play an important role, with evidence to suggest that families with more 'traditional' attitudes regard asking for professional help as a sign of failure.[397]

7.11 Carers may also find that there is no plateau to their caring role because of the degenerative nature of dementia. Continuous adjustments and adaptations may have to be made just at the point when the carer is starting to feel more competent and confident with what has just been achieved. Care requirements increase even though the carer's own health and resources may be diminishing, especially in the case of spouse or partner carers. Particular difficulties may arise when the person with dementia denies that there is anything wrong and refuses to accept any sort of additional help from paid care workers.

7.12 Many carers continue to see themselves as carers even when the person with dementia has moved into a care home, right up until the person with dementia dies. Writing about her experiences of caring for her mother with Alzheimer's disease, one carer notes that her "whole identity is shot through with being a carer. How can I stop thinking of myself as a carer just like that?"[398] However, some stop considering themselves as 'real' carers once the person with dementia is being cared for by others and then struggle to redefine their relationship with their loved one.[399]

Our approach

7.13 In Chapter 2 of this Report, we put forward the argument that the idea of solidarity is a key component in an ethical framework for the care and support of people with dementia. The concept of solidarity suggests that our response to the challenges presented by the increasingly common disorders leading to dementia should be one of 'fellow-travellers' where we seek to support and help one another. Families and friends demonstrate practical solidarity in the care and support they provide to people with dementia, whether this is given primarily out of love, compassion, duty, a desire to reciprocate past support, or a combination of all of these. We suggest that solidarity similarly urges us (as individuals, families, communities and through the state) to support carers in their own exercise of solidarity with those for whom they care.

7.14 Our ethical framework in Chapter 2 further emphasises the importance of giving close attention to the autonomy and well being of carers. This is partly because, in doing so, the autonomy and well-being of people with dementia are likely to be enhanced: a carer who feels properly supported and appreciated by others is likely in turn to be able to provide more supportive care and hence a better quality of life for people with dementia.[400] We also argue that autonomy should be seen in 'relational' terms: that is, that a person's sense of self and self-expression should be seen as being firmly grounded in their social and family networks. In addition, most people would wish that their carer's interests should be given considerable weight: their interests include their carer's interests. When autonomy is understood in these terms, then in order to support a person's autonomous wishes and values it will be necessary to support the whole family and social structure.

7.15 However, we also strongly advocate paying attention to the autonomy and well-being of carers because carers are people in their own right, whose own interests are important quite outside any associated benefit to the person with dementia. The very fact that carers are likely to neglect or

---

[397] Lawrence V, Murray J, Samsi K and Banerjee S (2008) Attitudes and support needs of Black Caribbean, south Asian and White British carers of people with dementia in the UK *British Journal of Psychiatry* **193**: 240–6.

[398] Healthy Living Blog (2008) Why caring makes you truly human, available at: www.saga.co.uk/health/healthyliving/blog/carer-diary/july-3-2008-why-caring-makes-you-truly-human.asp.

[399] Goldsteen M, Abma T, Oeseburg B *et al.* (2007) What is it to be a daughter? Identities under pressure in dementia care *Bioethics* **21(1)**: 1–12.

[400] Brodaty H, Green A and Koschera A (2003) Meta-analysis of psychosocial interventions for caregivers of people with dementia *Journal of the American Geriatric Society* **51**: 657–64.

even deny their own interests in order to promote the interests of the person for whom they care suggests that society, in the form of the professionals it employs, should have a concern for the interests of the carers, not only for the sake of the person with dementia but also for the sake of the carers themselves.

7.16 Alongside these ethical reasons for recognising the need to help and support carers, a purely pragmatic financial point should also be noted: if carers did not take on their roles to the extent they currently do, the financial impact on the state would be enormous, as the monetary value of the care provided by family and friends to people with dementia has been estimated at £5.4 billion in England alone.[401] Indeed, the point has been made that the only affordable way in the long term to provide care for people with dementia in both the developed and developing world is for support to be delivered through carers.[402]

7.17 We discussed in Chapter 4 how as individuals we could support people with dementia and their carers, both in our attitudes to and acceptance of dementia, and in some cases through practical voluntary help to those we know in our community who need support. We discuss below the role that the state and the voluntary sector, as providers and funders of health and social care services, can play in supporting carers. We consider help and support for carers first in terms of their role as carer and secondly in terms of their own personal needs as individuals.

Help and support for carers in their caring capacity

Joint support for the person with dementia and their carer

"Caring for a relative with dementia, of course, presents family carers with specific and complex problems. These can be exacerbated if their experience is framed within a medical model of care provision, a model which redefines the largely social consequences and which offers little in the way of helpful information."[403]

7.18 As we suggested earlier (see paragraphs 3.22 and 7.5), a diagnosis of possible dementia has implications that extend well beyond the individual receiving the diagnosis. Close family and friends, and especially the partner of the person with dementia, have to adjust to the ramifications for their own lives and come to terms with a shared future which may be very different from what they had all envisaged. We have already emphasised the need for appropriate information and follow-up for the person with dementia at the point of diagnosis (see paragraphs 3.25–3.29) and we note here the importance of ensuring that the information needs of carers, too, are met.

7.19 **An important implication both of our emphasis on solidarity and of our 'relational' approach to autonomy (see paragraph 7.14) is to emphasise that professional support should have a wide focus that includes helping family and friends to support the person with dementia, rather than being limited to an exclusive and direct focus on the person with dementia.** In much of medical care where people's ability to care for themselves and their mental capacity are not greatly affected, it is appropriate for health and social services to be focused almost exclusively on the patient or client. These models of service delivery may not be appropriate in dementia care, at least at some stages, where the major part of the care is delivered by the family or other carers. We highlight in Box 7.1 below the example of Admiral Nurses, whose approach is very much predicated on providing care to people with dementia *through* their existing family and other support networks.

---

[401] National Audit Office (2007) *Improving Services and Support for People with Dementia* (London: The Stationery Office), p9.

[402] See, for example, Ferri PF, Prince M, Brayne C *et al.* (2005) Global prevalence of dementia: a Delphi consensus study *The Lancet* **366**: 2112–7; Zaida A (2008) *Features and Challenges of Population Ageing: The European perspective* Policy Brief **March (1)** (Vienna: European Centre for Social Welfare Policy and Research).

[403] Gillies B (2000) Acting up: role ambiguity and the legal recognition of carers *Ageing and Society* **20**: 429–44.

> **Box 7.1: Example from practice – Admiral Nurses**
>
> Admiral Nurses are specialist mental health nurses who have experience in working with dementia. They support and work in partnership with people with dementia, their families, and their social networks. Admiral Nurses focus on working with carers, providing them with practical advice, emotional support and information. They visit carers and people with dementia in their own homes for as long as they are needed, working with carers throughout the duration of the person with dementia's illness. Admiral Nurses also deliver education and training in dementia care, and provide consultancy services to professionals working with people with dementia.
>
> Currently, Admiral Nurses operate in certain areas of England, including London, Kent, North East Lincolnshire, the West Midlands and the North West, and in North Wales.
>
> **More information:** www.fordementia.org.uk/admiral.htm.

Care partnerships

"In dementia care, there is much greater openness with carers (rightly or wrongly) than in other mental health contexts, and the need for partnership with family carers is widely recognised." Professor Bob Woods, consultation respondent

"Carers' skills must be recognised as such, working in partnership with a professional … so that the relationship of trust and honesty is built up." Dementia Services Development Centre (South East), Canterbury Christ Church University (Mrs Penny Hibberd, Admiral Nurse/ Senior Lecturer), consultation respondent

7.20 Carers will often know the person with dementia better than anyone else, and hence are likely to be well placed to advise on their particular support needs. However, they do not necessarily know about the nature or progression of dementia, nor what care interventions are possible. Support is therefore needed from professionals who do possess such knowledge. Conversely, health and social care professionals will be familiar with care planning, care provision and caregiving, but unfamiliar, at least initially, with the personal history, preferences and values of the person with dementia. As we note in Chapter 3 (see paragraph 3.12), it is therefore crucial that professionals and carers work together in genuine partnership, in order to ensure that people with dementia benefit from their joint expertise and joint knowledge.

7.21 Such a 'care partnership' should be founded on a basis of mutual respect for the different forms of knowledge of the different parties, and on the premise that all concerned are seeking to help the person live as well with their dementia as possible. We note in Chapter 3 (see paragraphs 3.30 and 3.31) the importance of ensuring that where formal services are available, they should be offered on a flexible basis, matched to the actual needs and wishes of those receiving them and to the support that carers are able and willing to offer.

7.22 As dementia progresses, the needs of both the person with dementia and their carer are likely to change significantly, and at some point it may become appropriate for the person to move into residential care, or for more formal support to be provided in the person's own home. It is imperative in such circumstances that the carer's continuing role is acknowledged, and that carers should be given opportunities to sustain whatever input they are able to contribute to the care for as long as they wish. When the level of formal support increases in this way, there should never be an 'all or nothing' assumption about the carer's desire to be involved or ability to cope. Some carers will wish to continue providing particular forms of care and support, such as washing their loved one's clothes, or taking in favourite food, even where the person with dementia is being cared for in a residential environment. Others may be happy to relinquish such tasks to others, but are still a rich source of information for those now providing day-to-day care for the person – for example through providing 'life-story books' to accompany the person into residential care.

The need to be trusted

> "To be cared for by others requires trust in the carer. It requires recognition of the carer as caring and of the importance of human community." *CARE, consultation respondent*

> "I think with something like dementia and something that is going to involve long term chronic deterioration in somebody, if you're going to get a good effective support for the patient you have to get the relatives – or whoever is going to do the caring – on board as soon as possible." *Carer, speaking on Healthtalkonline*[404]

7.23 The issue of trust is absolutely central in any caring relationship. Most carers provide a level of care that compromises their own health and well-being, and are concerned to help and support the person with dementia as much as they are able. This sense of duty is best captured in terms such as 'love', 'loyalty' and 'faithfulness', all of which are based on trust. Given this trust-based relationship between the person with dementia and their carer, there is an ethical imperative that professionals and care workers similarly start from a presumption of trust in the carer, in their good intentions and in their knowledge of the person with dementia (see also paragraph 3.12). Such trust will normally act to promote the autonomy of the person with dementia, understood in the relational sense highlighted in Chapter 2, as well as their well-being. **Unless there is evidence to the contrary, there should be a presumption of trust in carers by health and social care professionals and care workers. Such trust is a key part of any 'caring partnership', and without such trust it is highly unlikely that the person with dementia can be given the best possible support.** As we discussed in Chapter 6 (see paragraphs 6.39–6.45), there may sometimes be occasions when for a variety of reasons some carers do not act in the best interests of the person for whom they care, and when trust may not be appropriate. If any evidence emerges that trust in a particular carer is misplaced, the professional should act on that concern, in just the same way as they would act on concerns about other professionals or care workers. Where there are no such concerns, however, the caring partnership between carers and those paid to provide care can best be sustained, and the person with dementia best supported, through mutually trusting relationships.

Access to confidential information about the person with dementia

> "I was stunned that my doctor would not speak about my concerns ... I felt frightened about my husband's changes in behaviour ..." *Agnes Charnley, consultation respondent*

> "Patient confidentiality in our system has been distorted into a charter for secrecy, when staff feel confident to deny even useful or helpful information that would support the patient's care to other professionals or relatives." *Professor June Andrews, Director, Dementia Services Development Centre, University of Stirling, consultation respondent*

> "Sometimes families do not understand when you explain about confidentiality and they are frustrated not to be involved in consultations." *Anonymous consultation respondent*

7.24 The Mental Capacity Act Code of Practice stipulates that health and social care staff should ensure that they only disclose information about somebody who lacks capacity if it is in the best interests of the person concerned to do so, or when there is some other, lawful reason for them to do so.[405] A person granted a lasting power of attorney by the person with dementia is entitled to access

---

[404] Healthtalkonline is a charity website that lets users share experiences of health and illness, including dementia. An interview with a carer of a person with dementia is available at: www.healthtalkonline.org/Nerves_and_brain/Carers_of_people_with_dementia/People/Interview/829/Category/102/Clip/4010/confidentiality#confidentiality.

[405] Department of Constitutional Affairs (2007) *Mental Capacity Act Code of Practice* (London: The Stationery Office), paragraph 16.19.

information about the person, once they lack capacity, as long as the information is relevant to decisions they are able to make on behalf of the person.[406]

7.25 The Code of Practice, however, suggests that carers should not normally need to receive information from health and social care professionals about the person for whom they care, as such carers have their own knowledge of the person to guide their decisions. The Code notes that, despite the fact that a carer "will probably have good motives for wanting the information", the professionals "might feel strongly that disclosing the information would not be in the best interests of the person who lacks capacity and would amount to an invasion of their privacy."[407] The Code therefore appears to place an emphasis on withholding information, rather than sharing it, and fails to focus on why carers *could* need information in order to help them care properly for their loved one. The Scottish Code of Practice for professionals, on the other hand, simply states briefly: "It will be necessary to consider the adult's right to confidentiality and any previously expressed wishes about disclosure of information."[408]

7.26 **We strongly support the current legal position that when a person lacks capacity, their confidential information should only be disclosed to others where it is in the best interests of the person to do so. We believe, however, that the current guidance in the Mental Capacity Act Code of Practice on *when* it will be in a person's best interests to share information is too restrictive.** As we discuss in the context of diagnosis, dementia affects not only the individual with dementia, but also all those close to them, particularly those who take on the role of carer (see paragraph 3.22). When a person with dementia lacks capacity to make a particular decision about their health or welfare, it is clearly in their best interests that those involved in making the decision on their behalf have access to the necessary information and are appropriately supported. **Professionals should be made aware of the legitimate reasons why carers may ask for medical or other confidential information, and ordinarily start from the assumption that if a carer is involved in making a decision on behalf of the person with dementia, then they will need the same level of information as any other member of the care team. In short, carers should be provided with any information that it is necessary for them to know in order to carry out their caring role.**

Recommendation 14: We recommend that the Office of the Public Guardian, in conjunction with the Department of Health and regulatory bodies such as the General Medical Council and Nursing and Midwifery Council, should reconsider the guidance on confidentiality currently given in the Mental Capacity Act Code of Practice, and give greater weight to the reasons why carers may need access to confidential information when involved in making decisions as to the best interests of the person with dementia for whom they care.

Financial and social support

"Adequate financial and emotional support for carers should be offered to ease the stress and financial hardship incurred when looking after a person who is chronically ill." *AAC Research Unit, University of Stirling, consultation respondent*

7.27 Caring for a person with dementia is expensive. Costs incurred by carers include factors such as lost earnings, paying for respite and other care, and investing in adaptations and assistive technologies for the individual for whom they are caring.[409] The financial impact on the household may be even more dramatic in cases of early-onset dementia where the person with dementia is the primary

[406] *Ibid*, paragraph 16.9.
[407] *Ibid*, paragraph 16.30.
[408] Scottish Government (2007) *Adults with Incapacity (Scotland) Act 2000 Code of Practice: For persons authorised to carry out medical treatment or research under Part 5 of the Act* (Edinburgh: The Scottish Government), paragraph 1.6.7.
[409] See paragraphs 6.5 to 6.12 for discussion on assistive technologies.

breadwinner in the household at the time of diagnosis. Although the benefit system in the UK includes a Carer's Allowance, this is limited to those who spend at least 35 hours a week caring for a person who receives either Attendance Allowance or Disability Living Allowance, and these benefits in turn are difficult to obtain without a formal diagnosis.[410] Given that over half of those with dementia do not currently obtain such a diagnosis,[411] many carers will find it difficult to obtain financial support for this reason alone. In addition, carer organisations such as Carers UK highlight how many carers miss out on welfare benefits to which they are potentially entitled.[412]

7.28 A carer's needs for support are not limited to financial matters, but also encompass emotional and practical support. Carers are entitled by law to a 'carer's assessment' by social services to see if they are entitled to support in their caring role, such as help in the house, adaptations, emotional support or a break from caring.[413] In a report by the House of Commons Committee of Public Accounts, however, it was noted that between half and two-thirds of all carers do not receive this assessment. In its recommendations, the Committee held that the Department of Health should "emphasise to local health organisations and their social care partners that they need to develop an action plan which gives priority to assessing and meeting the needs of carers."[414]

Box 7.2: Example from practice – support and education for carers

Interaction training project

As part of the **Forth Valley Dementia Project**, the Dementia Services Development Centre in Stirling has developed a course to help relatives, carers and care support workers in the Falkirk area understand dementia better and improve their interaction with those for whom they care.

The course gives participants an opportunity to share experiences and consider practical ways of responding to the person with dementia. It helps participants understand what dementia is and what changes occur in the brains of those affected. It also focuses on ways of communicating and how to anticipate and deal with challenging forms of behaviour. It ends with a practical session that involves working with people to maximise communication, understand behaviours better and strengthen relationships.

More information: Dementia Services Development Centre (2008) *The Forth Valley Dementia Project* (Stirling: DSDC), p13.

Caring with Confidence

Caring with Confidence is a Department of Health backed initiative that offers free knowledge and skills-based learning for carers in England. This new programme, which is part of the Government's New Deal for Carers and the National Carers' Strategy, offers support and help to carers with particular emphasis on those who provide care on a daily basis but have difficulty finding out how to access the services and benefits available to them. It also aims to help carers to look at the essential aspects of looking after someone and how to communicate effectively with other people to help support their needs.

Carers can choose how they access the Caring with Confidence programme, either by attending face-to-face group sessions, completing self-study workbooks, accessing online sessions or a combination of all three. As part of the programme, special sessions for carers of people with dementia will be provided by the Alzheimer's Society in late 2009 in Sussex, Somerset, Devon and Hampshire.

More information: www.caringwithconfidence.net/ and http://alzheimers.org.uk/site/scripts/press_article.php?articleID=345.

7.29 Some carers find it very difficult to ask for the help that they need in order to cope with the situation in which they find themselves, especially where their adult identity has been based on a solid foundation of competence, capability and independence. It may take time for carers to realise that they are not coping, especially if they are making every effort to do so, and sometimes they may see asking for help as an admission of failure. Even once they have acknowledged the need for outside help, they may have difficulty in accessing it, for example because of a lack of knowledge about how the 'system' works.

---

[410] For example, Attendance Allowance and Disability Living Allowance application forms require details of the person's illness and any treatment that they receive.

[411] National Audit Office (2007) *Improving Services and Support for People with Dementia* (London: The Stationery Office), p7.

[412] See, for example, Carers UK (2005) *Caring and Pensioner Poverty: A report on older carers, employment and benefits* (London: Carers UK).

[413] s1 Carers and Disabled Children Act 2000 in England and Wales; s9 Community Care and Health (Scotland) Act 2002; s1 Carers and Direct Payments (Northern Ireland) Act 2002.

[414] House of Commons Committee of Public Accounts (2008) *Improving Services and Support for People with Dementia* (London: The Stationery Office), p5.

7.30 Our emphasis on solidarity highlights society's responsibility to support people with dementia and their carers. This responsibility extends to informing carers, openly and systematically, of the social and financial support to which they are entitled: support should not only be available to those who know enough about the system and have sufficient persistence to assert their rights. We again commend the proposed role of a dementia care adviser or similar (see paragraph 3.27) who should be well placed to ensure that carers of people with dementia are better informed about their entitlements. We reiterate that a timely diagnosis (see paragraph 3.18) is also important for carers, given that without such a diagnosis carers will experience significant difficulty in obtaining the help and support they themselves need.

The help and support carers need as individuals

7.31 We have already argued that carers are individuals in their own right, and have a moral right to be treated as such (see paragraphs 2.40, 2.41 and 7.15). Carers therefore have rights for their own sake, and also, crucially, a need for support in a variety of areas.

Maintaining one's own identity

"[I] gave up teaching, singing, all things that gave me my identity." *Agnes Charnley, consultation respondent*

"Those caring need … the opportunity to meet and talk about other topics, so that their whole life does not revolve around dementia." *Hazel Simpson, consultation respondent*

7.32 As we noted in paragraph 7.7, it takes time and reflection to acknowledge and assume for oneself both the 'role' and 'identity' of being a carer, even though that role or function may be obvious to others. Some carers may even reject their 'carer' identity altogether, and continue to see themselves as, for example, a daughter and not a carer.[415] Many types of adjustments are required before one can do so, especially where a diagnosis of dementia is delayed or absent.

7.33 It was also clear from our consultation that many carers face difficulties in maintaining their *own* identity when caring for their relative: in taking on the identity of a carer they risk losing aspects of what it meant to be themselves. It is therefore crucial that mechanisms are in place in order to allow carers to hold on to their own identity, for example through access to regular respite services in order to give them free space to be themselves and pursue their interests outside their caring role. We suggested in paragraphs 7.20 and 7.21 that carers should be seen as 'care partners' in their role of supporting the person with dementia. As a 'partner' in care, the carer should be able to feel that they are not solely responsible, and that it is legitimate for them to have some time to themselves while others provide the necessary care for their loved one.

> **Box 7.3: Example from practice – Falkirk 'home from home' service**
>
> The 'home from home' service is part of Falkirk Council's Joint Dementia Initiative (JDI) and involves individuals in the community welcoming people with dementia into their homes on either one or two days a week. People with dementia (living on their own or living with carers) are collected by the home owner or a member of the JDI staff and taken to the person's home. The people with dementia then spend the day choosing what they would like for meals, helping prepare the meal and carrying out other tasks such as washing the dishes. The focus is on helping people with dementia experience everyday life, from eating meals together to spending time chatting or maybe doing a crossword together, rather than attending a more institutional form of care such as a day centre. The choice of activities is up to those who attend, and the home owner and member of staff have plenty of opportunity to spend time with each person.
>
> **More information available at:** http://dementia.stir.ac.uk/pdffolder/FVDP-HomeFromHome.pdf. **Contact details:** Joint Dementia Initiative Falkirk Council, telephone: 01324 501730.

---

[415] Goldsteen M, Abma T, Oeseburg B *et al.* (2007) What is it to be a daughter? Identities under pressure in dementia care *Bioethics* **21(1)**: 1–12.

> **Box 7.4: Example from practice – carers' leisure pass**
>
> **The Princess Royal Trust Salford Carers' Centre** is piloting a carers' leisure pass, which gives carers unlimited access to council swimming, gym and leisure facilities. Use of the pass is monitored, and if it is not used for a continuous period of two months, the Carers' Centre is informed and the carer is contacted to check if they are well.
>
> More information: The Princess Royal Trust for Carers (2008) *Putting People First Without Putting Carers Second* (Essex: The Princess Royal Trust for Carers), p29, available at: http://static.carers.org/files/putting-people-first-09-individual-pages-4069.pdf.

Counselling

> "I didn't realise I was grieving. I thought you only grieved when someone was dead, and my wife isn't dead! I didn't know grieving could start with the diagnosis of a chronic illness."
> *Anonymous participant on family carers' course*

7.34 For some carers, the option of counselling sessions may help them to understand and come to terms with some of their emotions, including possible feelings of guilt, anger and grief.[416] Counselling may be particularly necessary where the carer and the person with dementia have had a past emotional relationship that has been troubled or distant, although the need for counselling support may arise in any long-term caring relationship. By providing a 'safe place' where emotions can be explored in a non-judgmental way, counselling can help carers to come to terms with their own emotions about caring; support them in particular difficult situations in their caring role; and in some cases help them come to terms with the idea that other options of care should be considered.

Considering one's own interests

7.35 It is also essential that carers are supported in considering their *own* interests, as well as those for whom they care. In Chapter 5, we highlighted how, in making a particular decision for a person who lacks capacity to make that decision for themselves, others are legally required to act in that person's 'best interests'. At first sight, this suggests that the interests of the person with dementia should always be placed above those surrounding them. Yet, as we note above (see paragraph 7.14), interests are often complex and intertwined. In a family, it will rarely be the case that a single person's interests always take priority: rather some consideration will be given to everyone's interests and some degree of compromise found.

7.36 The Mental Capacity Act reflects this reality in its broad approach to 'best interests'. A determination of a person's best interests is not limited simply to what, in the abstract, might seem best for their personal welfare or well-being, but also includes consideration of factors such as their beliefs and values (see Box 5.2) and other factors they might have taken into account themselves. In many cases this will include strong concern for the welfare of others in their family. Moreover, any determination of a person's 'best interests' is inevitably limited by practical constraints, including finance and the availability of particular forms of support; and there can be no legal or ethical duty to continue caring where this is no longer physically or emotionally viable.

7.37 However, it may be very difficult for a carer genuinely to consider their own interests alongside those of the person for whom they care, even if they know that this is what the person with dementia would have wished. **Professionals such as doctors, nurses, clinical psychologists and social workers have an important role to play in supporting carers explicitly to consider their own needs and interests when weighing up difficult decisions, particularly around future care options.**

---

[416] See, for example, Alzheimer's Society (2008) *Counselling: How can it help?* Factsheet 445 (London: Alzheimer's Society), available at http://alzheimers.org.uk/factsheet/445; Gibson J (2009) Living with loss *Mental Health Practice* **12(5)**: 22–4.

7.38 It is also crucial for professionals to be aware of how carers' own needs may change significantly, to the extent that their needs may in fact be greater than those of the person for whom they care. This may particularly arise where one elderly spouse is caring for the other. Where the carer's own cognitive abilities are beginning to become impaired, professionals need to be alert both as to the carer's own needs and to the extent to which they are still capable of making decisions as a carer for the person with dementia, for example in terms of understanding the risks involved in day-to-day care. In situations where the carer is a long-standing partner, the relationship between the person with dementia and the carer may be fundamentally important to the well-being of both. In such difficult situations, it will be crucial for professionals to consider both the individual and shared priorities of care for the couple.

Chapter 8

Research

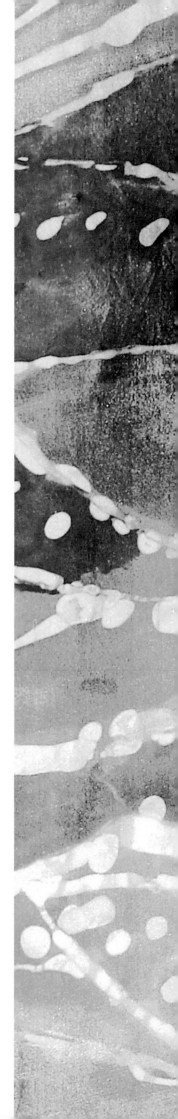

Chapter 8 – Research

Introduction

8.1   This Chapter will focus on two specific ethical issues posed by research into dementia. First, it will discuss how research should be prioritised, given both the 'Cinderella status' of dementia and the inherent tension between the longer-term and unpredictable aim of seeking cures and the shorter-term and perhaps more immediate goal of enhancing quality of life. Secondly, it will consider the particular difficulties which arise when involving people with cognitive impairment in research studies.

How should research be prioritised?

"Surveys of carers show that what is wanted is a better understanding of the causes, so they might become preventable. Surveys of dementia sufferers indicate that there is more concern regarding quality of life issues." *Anonymous consultation respondent*

"… the emphasis of resource allocation, prioritisation, performance targets, research funding, education and training has all been skewed towards higher tech treatments and 'sexier' conditions such as cancer or ischaemic heart disease which affect younger people and away from the needs of older people with incurable long term conditions." *British Geriatrics Society, consultation respondent*

8.2   While there have been major advances in recent years in dementia research, the 2007 report *Dementia UK*, produced by the London School of Economics and King's College London for the Alzheimer's Society, highlighted the relatively low priority given to dementia research compared with that devoted to other diseases. A survey of research papers on long-term conditions published since 2002 demonstrated that while 23.5 per cent were concerned with cancer and 17.6 per cent with cardiovascular diseases, only 1.4 per cent focused on dementia.[417] In June 2009, the UK Clinical Research Network listed 104 trials for dementias or other neurodegenerative diseases being set up or currently recruiting, compared with 218 for cardiovascular diseases and 383 for cancer.[418] Similar differences are found in the levels of public funding for medical research: figures on combined research funding by the English Department of Health and Medical Research Council published in response to parliamentary questions cited a total of £32.4 million spent in 2007–8 on dementia, compared with £248.2 million the same year on cancer[419] – a distinction much criticised by organisations such as the Alzheimer's Research Trust.[420]

8.3   Before commenting further on the implications of these figures, however, we would first like to consider what research into dementia should be trying to achieve. We identify below six broad areas of potential research into dementia, all of which received considerable support in our public consultation.

8.4   **Basic science research**: working to understand both the mechanisms of normal ageing and the mechanisms which lead to the death of brain cells and hence brain atrophy. As the Academy of Medical Sciences highlighted in their response to us, the precise mechanisms causing neurodegeneration are still unclear, despite identification that a number of proteins, such as

---

[417]   Knapp M and Prince M (King's College London and London School of Economics) (2007) *Dementia UK* (London: Alzheimer's Society), pxv.

[418]   Figures correct as at 9 July 2009, see: http://public.ukcrn.org.uk/Search/Portfolio.aspx.

[419]   House of Commons *Hansard*, 16 December 2008, c677W, available at: www.publications.parliament.uk/pa/cm200809/cmhansrd/cm081216/text/81216w0033.htm#08121714000065.

[420]   Alzheimer's Research Trust website, available at: www.alzheimers-research.org.uk/info/statistics/.

amyloid, tau and the presenilins, and the gene ApoE4 all have important roles.[421] Until we have a better understanding of what role these particular hallmarks of the different dementias play in the development of the disease, we will be limited in our ability to identify new targets for possible drug treatments. Basic science research is also required to understand the reason why ageing of the brain leads to dementia in some people and not in others, especially given that Alzheimer-type pathology has been found in the post-mortem examination of brains of people who exhibited no symptoms of dementia during their lifetime.[422] Basic science research in other areas involved in normal ageing, such as sensory impairments, is of particular relevance for people with dementia: we currently know very little either about how these impairments contribute to the effect of the person's dementia on their mood and behaviour or about how the pathology of the dementia itself may itself compound sensory losses.[423]

8.5 **Development of treatments.** The primary aim of much current research into dementia treatments is to find strategies which will limit, and ultimately halt, the damage to the brain, for example by research into techniques to reverse the accumulation of amyloid in the brain. We have already noted in Chapter 1 that, given the way our brains 'age' even without dementia, the idea of a simple 'cure' for dementia is misleading (see paragraph 1.30). Moreover, for people living with dementia, the most important aspect of their condition will generally be the effect of the dementia on their day-to-day life (both in terms of cognitive and behavioural changes) and the rate at which their difficulties increase. Research therefore needs to focus on possible treatments to delay or limit the effects of the underlying pathology on daily life, as well as tackling the pathology, such as the accumulation of amyloid, itself. One of the criticisms levelled against NICE's decision to recommend only limited NHS access to the cholinesterase inhibitors in England and Wales, for example, is NICE's alleged failure to pay sufficient attention to the personal experiences of many people with dementia and their carers, who reported significant improvements, albeit for a temporary period, in their quality of life.[424] Moreover, it is important that research addresses drug development for all the various different types of dementia: the UK Age Research Forum, for example, highlighted the lack of work in this area for several diseases leading to dementia, including vascular dementia.[425]

8.6 **Prevention,** or at least strategies to delay the onset of dementia. Work in this area would include research into genetic predispositions to dementia; long-term cohort studies (drawing from across all ethnic groups) which aim to increase understanding of the influence of lifetime risk factors such as environmental influences, diet and lifestyle; and research into 'neuroprotective' strategies and treatments, such as the effect of cognitive activity earlier in life on developing a 'cognitive reserve' against dementia.

8.7 **Social science research** seeking a better understanding of issues such as:

- the experience of living with dementia, both as a person with a diagnosis of dementia and as a family member or carer;
- how quality of life is affected throughout the course of a person's dementia;

[421] Academy of Medical Sciences, responding to the Working Party's consultation.

[422] Neuropathology Group of the Medical Research Council Cognitive Function and Ageing Study (2001) Pathological correlates of late-onset dementia in a multicentre, community-based population in England and Wales *The Lancet* **357**: 169–75.

[423] Uhlmann RF, Larson EB, Koepsell TD, Rees TS and Duckert LG (1991) Visual impairment and cognitive dysfunction in Alzheimer's Disease *Journal of General Internal Medicine* **6**: 126–32; Pham TQ, Kifley A, Mitchell P and Wang JJ (2006) Relation of age-related macular degeneration and cognitive impairment in an older population *Gerontology* **52**: 353–8.

[424] Alzheimer's Society statement *Access to drugs*, available at: http://62.216.236.229/site/scripts/documents.php?categoryID=200264; see also Foresight (2008) *Mental Capital and Well-being: Making the most of ourselves in the 21st century – final project report* (London: Government Office for Science), p212, where it is argued that the indirect effect on carers, in terms of their well-being and productivity, is not properly considered in the current process for determining the cost-effectiveness of drugs.

[425] The UK Age Research Forum, responding to the Working Party's consultation.

- the role of stigma in affecting how people with dementia cope with their condition, and how stigma can best be challenged;
- how people can best be supported to 'live well' with their dementia, including the effect of the 'small things' of life such as the courtesy and respect with which others treat them in everyday matters;
- the most effective approaches to educating and supporting professionals and care workers in their understanding of and response to people with dementia;
- how best to educate and support those providing paid or unpaid care in responding to the ethical challenges they face on a daily basis; and
- the potential effect of wider environmental and social changes, such as attempts to make buildings and services more 'dementia-friendly', on the daily lives of people with dementia and those close to them.

8.8 **Care to improve the lives of people with dementia now,** including:

- comparative health services research on what is effective in caring for and supporting people with dementia; what forms of support are most cost-effective; the factors that affect the transferability of existing models of good practice; and the factors affecting the speed with which developments in the evidence base spread into day-to-day practice;
- nursing research on how to manage physical care needs appropriately in dementia;
- the use of technology to help people retain independence for longer; and
- development of more non-drug treatments and strategies to help people with dementia and their carers cope with difficult moods and behaviours.[426]

8.9 A sixth category, that of **'translational research'**, aims to support the outcomes of one or more of the research targets above: for example the encouragement of early trials to enable swifter transfer from laboratory to clinical practice; the development of biomarkers, with the long-term aim of distinguishing between different dementias at an earlier stage and improving clinical trials by providing more reliable markers of how the disease is progressing; the creation of 'clinical cohorts' to facilitate longitudinal research; and the development of models to investigate the drivers of disease.

8.10 In their responses to our public consultation, major research funding bodies, such as the UK Age Research Forum (representing the views of almost 30 funding bodies), the Wellcome Trust, the Medical Research Council and the Economic and Social Research Council were in agreement that all of these broad research areas were important and required attention. It was noted that, in general, preventative research receives a relatively small proportion of research funding, and that this holds true for dementia.[427] Indeed, analysis carried out by UK Clinical Research Collaboration in 2006 suggested that just 0.3 per cent of all neurological research related to prevention.[428] The importance of work in this field was underlined to us by the UK Age Research Forum, who commented that it will "not be sustainable" in the future simply to try to ameliorate symptoms and provide long-term care: if the average onset of dementia is not delayed, there will simply be too many people with dementia for the system to cope. As we have already noted (see paragraph 1.29), 'preventative' strategies that result overall in people living longer may not reduce the numbers experiencing dementia, as increased age itself is a significant risk factor for dementia.

---

[426] The guidelines published in 2006 by SIGN highlighted a number of areas in this category where the research base is currently far from adequate, including research on alternatives to drug treatment, the role of physical exercise in maintaining independent living, how to treat pain in dementia, effective interventions for "repetitive vocalisations" and the most effective way to prevent falls in dementia: SIGN (2006) *Management of Patients with Dementia: A national clinical guideline* (Edinburgh: SIGN), paragraph 6.4.

[427] The UK Age Research Forum, responding to the Working Party's consultation.

[428] UK Clinical Research Collaboration (2006) *UK Health Research Analysis* (London: UK Clinical Research Collaboration), p28.

However, such strategies may still be effective if, overall, they reduce the number of years of living with the more disabling aspects of dementia, even if the total number of people developing dementia before they die increases.[429]

8.11 While direct figures as to the amount spent on research into care models in dementia are not readily available, the UK Clinical Research Collaboration research cited above demonstrated that for the larger category of neurological research as a whole, only 0.3 per cent of expenditure was devoted to health services research.[430] The British Geriatrics Society suggested to us that one cause of the low levels of funding in this area of research is the emphasis placed in the Research Assessment Exercise (on which government funding for universities is partly based) on publications in high-impact journals. This may make it difficult for departments of gerontology or old age psychiatry to compete on equal terms with those concerned with basic science research; indeed, the Society argues that it is "difficult for academic departments of geriatric medicine or old age psychiatry to survive let alone flourish" in this funding environment.[431]

8.12 It was clear from our public consultation that many people, especially those with direct first-hand experience of dementia, felt that more research effort needed to be focused on different models of care with the aim of improving the quality of life of people who are living with dementia now.[432] Indeed, it has been noted in the context of the English dementia strategy that a key gap in current research evidence is research relating to longer-term outcomes of particular types of care models.[433] Some of the key elements in the strategy itself, such as dementia care advisers and improved end of life care for people with dementia, are in fact recommendations for 'demonstrator projects', subject to future evaluation. Concern was also expressed to us, for example by members of the Bradford Dementia Group, that even where research evidence *does* exist that particular forms of care and therapy are beneficial for people with dementia, there appears to be little impetus to ensure that they are implemented.[434] Exploring why this is the case, and what models of care are readily transferable between different geographical areas and services, is a further important research question.

8.13 It should also be noted that different types of research have the capacity to benefit different groups. Prevention and cure both seek primarily to benefit future generations, while research focused on quality of care has the potential to benefit people with dementia in the near future. There are also very different degrees of uncertainty involved: while research relating to quality of life and care is likely to produce some benefit (even if hard to measure), no-one can at present predict whether current research targets within basic science will turn out to be blind alleys or, alternatively, may transform the research landscape. Do we 'bet' on the enormous benefits to be obtained by developing either effective preventative strategies or a cure, or do we prioritise readily achievable improvements in day-to-day care and support?

---

[429] Brayne C, Gao Lu, Dewey M and Matthews FE (2006) Dementia before death in ageing societies: the promise of prevention and the reality *PLoS Medicine* **3(10)**: e397; Jagger C, Matthews R, Lindesay J *et al.* (2009) The effect of dementia trends and treatments on longevity and disability: a simulation model based on the MRC Cognitive Function and Ageing Study (MRC CFAS) *Age and Ageing* **38**: 319–25.

[430] UK Clinical Research Collaboration (2006) *UK Health Research Analysis* (London: UK Clinical Research Collaboration), p28.

[431] British Geriatrics Society, responding to the Working Party's consultation. The House of Commons Science and Technology Committee has raised similar concerns about the perceived impact of particular journals within the Research Assessment Exercise (RAE) process, and reminded RAE panels that they are obliged to judge the quality of individual articles, not the reputation of the journal in which they are published: House of Commons Science and Technology Committee (2004) *Tenth report*, part 9, paragraph 210, available at: www.publications.parliament.uk/pa/cm200304/cmselect/cmsctech/399/39912.htm#a54.

[432] Nuffield Council on Bioethics (2009) *Dementia: Ethical issues – summary of public consultation* (London: Nuffield Council on Bioethics), Q29.

[433] Burns A and Robert P (2009) The National Dementia strategy in England: a 'smorgasbord' of evidence, economics and obligation *British Medical Journal* **338**: 614.

[434] Working Party's fact-finding meeting with the Bradford Dementia Group, 29 July 2008.

8.14 A final important issue in connection with research into both treatment and care is the outcome measures used. We have noted in paragraphs 1.5 and 8.5 that the availability of medicines within the NHS is linked with their cost-effectiveness, and that this calculation in turn will be strongly dependent on the way that the effectiveness of the medicine is measured. A European taskforce recently reviewed the various outcomes or endpoints used in research into mild, moderate and severe Alzheimer's disease, and recommended that "cognition and function" should be the two primary outcomes in research into symptomatic treatment of mild and moderate disease, while factors such as "time to reach a specified incapacity scale, entry to institutional care, number of admissions to hospital, need for home help, level of satisfaction, lack of a basic ADL [activity of daily living] and onset of behavioural disorders" are all relevant outcomes in severe Alzheimer's disease.[435] While the increasing focus on factors such as levels of satisfaction and the person's ability to function in everyday life is strongly to be welcomed, further research is needed in this area into how outcome measures can reflect, as accurately as possible, the extent to which both medicines and non-pharmacological treatments and services genuinely help the person to live well with their dementia. Such research also needs to go beyond Alzheimer's disease to cover all dementias.

Our approach to research priorities

8.15 A constant theme running throughout this Report has been the impact, worldwide, of the growing prevalence of dementia. As more people in both developed and developing countries live to greater ages, so the likelihood of developing dementia at the end of life increases. Dementia, as currently experienced, imposes a significant economic burden both on families and the state, and we have cited above the view of the UK Age Research Forum that the systems currently in place to support people with dementia (imperfect as they are) will simply not be able to cope in the future. In our own ethical framework, set out in Chapter 2, we argue that an appropriate, and ethical, response to the increasing challenge posed by dementia is that of solidarity: accepting a mutual responsibility for supporting people with dementia. A key aspect of this solidarity must also be a commitment to supporting research into dementia, with the aim of minimising the effect of dementia on all concerned.

8.16 We are aware of the difficulties inherent in making comparisons between the funding available for research into dementia and funding available for other conditions. Funding comes from many different sources, including charitable funding, which in some cases will be heavily dependent on individuals' willingness to donate; research does not take place in 'silos', and a breakthrough in one area of science may turn out to have major implications for another apparently unconnected area; the value of putting large resources into an area of research depends on the current state of knowledge and techniques; and thus the quality of research is not related solely to levels of funding. Nevertheless, the low levels of funding for dementia research in comparison with many other conditions is striking in the light of the numbers affected, the extent of disability resulting from the condition and the economic impact of the condition.[436] It seems unlikely that dementia research is receiving a fair or appropriate proportion of funding in medical research.

---

[435] Vellas B, Andrieu S, Sampaio C, Coley N and Wilcock G (2008) Endpoints for trials in Alzheimer's disease: a European taskforce consensus *Lancet Neurology* **7**: 436–50.

[436] See, for example, Lowin A, Knapp M and McCrone P (2001) Alzheimer's disease in the UK: comparative evidence on cost of illness and volume of health services research funding *International Journal of Geriatric Psychiatry* **16**: 1143–8. See also World Health Organization (2008) *Global Burden of Disease 2004* (Geneva: WHO Press), table 13, where dementia is cited as the fourth highest cause of 'burden of disease' (measured in terms of lost years of full health) in high-income countries, after unipolar depressive disorders, ischaemic heart disease and cerebrovascular disease.

8.17 We are struck by the fact that the major research funding bodies within the UK do not appear to have explicit policies according to which they allocate funds between different conditions, focusing rather on research excellence and the 'importance' of the topic.[437] While it is clearly appropriate that funding bodies support important and high-quality research, criteria such as these do not, alone, ensure a just distribution between the needs of different parts of the population. **We believe that major research funders should be more explicit as to how they divide their research funds between areas of research that have the capacity to benefit very different groups of the population. Given the social and economic impact of dementia, we believe that a more explicit approach to research priorities would be likely to lead to significant increases in research funding for dementia. If such an increase were not to be matched by research applications of the necessary high standard, then active steps should be taken to develop and promote research capacity in the relevant areas.**

Recommendation 15: We recommend that the major research funders develop, and articulate, a reasoned basis for the division of their research funds between areas of research which have the capacity to benefit very different groups of the population. We further recommend that, if necessary, they take active steps to promote and sustain the creation of research communities capable of carrying out high-quality research.

8.18 On the question of how funding should be prioritised *within* dementia research, we agree with the major funding bodies that all the types of research into dementia outlined in paragraphs 8.4–8.9 above are important and no one type of research can be highlighted as having priority over others. We would, however, make the following observations:

- There appears to be widespread agreement that research into the effectiveness and transferability of different models of care and support for people with dementia is relatively neglected. Yet research into these areas is crucial if people are to be supported to live well with dementia. This is particularly important given that the prospect of a real cure for dementia is highly elusive (see paragraphs 1.30, 1.31 and 8.5).
- There are also widespread concerns about the outcome measures used when assessing the effectiveness or cost-effectiveness of a particular treatment or service, as evidenced, for example, by the challenges to the NICE decision on cholinesterase inhibitors.
- It is crucial to understand better how people with dementia and their carers live with dementia, how dementia affects them throughout the course of the disease, and how their quality of life could be improved throughout those stages. Social research in this area is an essential starting point for both the research into care models and the development of sensitive outcome measures described above. More research into the effects of stigma and how stigma can best be challenged would also be highly valuable.
- We highlight throughout this Report how all those involved in caring for people with dementia need better access to ethical education and support in order to respond to the ethical problems they encounter on a daily basis. Further research is required on how best to achieve this aim, encompassing both research into the content of the teaching, and appropriate educational teaching methods.
- Research into non-Alzheimer's dementias lags far behind that into Alzheimer's disease.
- Research into preventative strategies appears to receive too low a priority.

---

[437] The Medical Research Council, for example, states that "The main factors in funding decisions are research excellence – i.e. the likelihood of major advances in knowledge – and the importance of the topic", see: www.mrc.ac.uk/About/Strategy/Principles/index.htm.

Recommendation 16: We recommend that relevant research funders consider ways in which the level of funding for dementia research could be increased in the following areas: health services research into how people with dementia and their carers can best be supported to live well, how mainstream services can best be adapted to their needs, and how good practice can more readily be implemented; more meaningful outcome measures for assessing the effect of particular forms of treatment or service; research into how best to improve the provision of support for ethical decision making; all forms of research for the non-Alzheimer's dementias; and research into preventative strategies.

Recommendation 17: We particularly highlight the importance of social research in providing an evidence base to underpin better ways of supporting people with dementia and their carers. We recommend that funding bodies such as the Economic and Social Research Council, in partnership with others, take active steps to encourage further research into issues such as how people live with dementia, the nature of their experience and the quality of their lives; how stigma can best be challenged; and how those working in health and social care can best be supported in providing care which genuinely respects the personhood of everyone with dementia.

8.19 We also note, and welcome, a number of recent developments throughout the UK, which seek to promote research into dementia and encourage closer links between research and clinical practice. These include: the 'research summit' promised for July 2009 by the English dementia strategy; the development of clinical networks such as the National Institute for Health Research's Dementias and Neurodegenerative Diseases Research Network (DeNDRoN), the Scottish Dementia Research Network, the Dementias and Neurodegenerative Diseases Research Network in Wales (NEURODEM Cymru) and the Northern Ireland Clinical Research Network in dementia;[438] and the funding by the National Institute of Health Research of dementia-specific programmes such as 'EvIDem' (Evidence Based Interventions in Dementia)[439] and SHIELD (Support at Home – Interventions to Enhance Life with Dementia).[440]

Who should be involved in research?

Choosing to be involved in research

"I feel like I'm doing something not only interesting but I think something that's needed."[441]

"People with dementia, sometimes even quite moderately severe dementia, often have an idea as to whether or not they wish to participate in research, and it is very important that they are consulted." *Professor Gordon Wilcock, consultation respondent*

8.20 Individuals with the capacity to make their own decisions as to whether or not to be involved in research may be involved only if they give consent. As with consent to treatment, consent to research participation must be sufficiently informed and given voluntarily if it is to be legally valid. Research participants are entitled to withdraw from research at any time, with no obligation to give a reason.

8.21 People choose to participate in research, including research related to dementia, for a wide range of reasons. They may wish to access an experimental treatment before it is generally available in the hope that they will benefit. They may have altruistic reasons for participating, even where they do not expect to benefit personally. They may also find that the process of taking part in research

---

[438] For more information, see: www.dendron.org.uk/about/index.html; www.ukcrn.org.uk/index/networks/uk_wide.html; www.wales.nhs.uk/sites3/page.cfm?orgid=580&pid=14713; www.nicrn.hscni.net/themednetworks.aspx.

[439] See: www.evidem.org.uk/.

[440] See: www.nelft-rd.co.uk/research/current_research/shield/index.php.

[441] Henderson CS (1998) *Partial View: An Alzheimer's journal* (Dallas: Southern Methodist University Press), p63, on participating in research.

(such as extra attention from health professionals and the sense of being involved) is enjoyable or beneficial.

8.22 The ability of people with dementia to make their own decisions (if necessary with plenty of support) as to whether or not they wish to participate in research should not be underestimated. Nor should it be forgotten that a person's capacity may fluctuate significantly: for example, people with dementia may have 'good' and 'bad' times of day and may be able to make their own decision if approached at the right time and in the right way. A person with dementia should receive all possible support to help them make their own decision about involvement in a particular piece of research, at the time the decision is required. We will return to this point in paragraphs 8.39 and 8.45, when we consider the way information about research is presented.

The aims of research

8.23 The main aim of medical research is to gain knowledge that, it is hoped, will benefit people in the future. There is a distinction between research that has the potential to benefit those who take part and that which does not. An example of research that may benefit those taking part is a trial comparing current treatment with a novel treatment. An example of research which does not have the potential to benefit those taking part is basic science research concerned with a better understanding of dementia that is unlikely to result in any improvement in management for many years.

8.24 One concern which is often raised when considering the consent requirements for research (whether or not the person has capacity to consent for themselves) is the extent to which people participating in research may not properly understand these distinctions and hence may participate primarily in the hope of personal benefit where this is inappropriate.[442] This may be a problem particularly where the two paradigms of research described above have the potential to become intertwined: for example in the case of early research into new treatments, where participants are bound to hope there is some chance the treatment will help them directly, even when they understand that the outcome is unknown and that in any case they may unknowingly receive a placebo or an existing treatment rather than the new treatment.

Involving people with impaired capacity in research

8.25 Where individuals do not have the capacity to make their own decision about participating in research, and where the research is not likely to benefit the participant, several different approaches have been suggested:

Prohibition on involvement in research

"Avoiding research on participants who lack capacity through dementia is prejudicial to the elderly and to the mentally and neurologically unwell and is in our view unethical."
Alzheimer's Research Trust, consultation respondent

"I don't think it is right to involve anyone in research without their informed consent."
Hazel Simpson, consultation respondent

8.26 At one end of the spectrum, it could be argued that people should *never* be involved in research if they lack the capacity to make this decision for themselves. Concerns, for example, are expressed about people being made to participate in research when it simply cannot be known whether they

---

442 Appelbaum PS, Roth LH, Lidz CW, Benson P and Winslade W (1987) False hopes and best data: consent to research and the therapeutic misconception *Hastings Center Report* **17(2)**: 20–4.

wish to do so or not.[443] Critics of this position argue that such an approach, if applied more widely, would prevent much beneficial research in other areas where participants cannot give consent for themselves, preventing improvements in the care of babies, emergency treatment in Accident and Emergency departments and care for people in comas. It is also argued that it is positively unethical to exclude people from research who are not able to give valid consent, as whole sections of the population may thus be excluded from the benefits that research may bring.

8.27 Moreover, as highlighted above, many people with dementia do show positive willingness and enthusiasm for being involved in research, even if their understanding of the precise details of the research project concerned may not be sufficient for a legally valid consent to be obtained. As one carer commented: "[My mother] would be quite cross to think that she could not take part, because she could no longer consent herself."

Giving consent in advance

"I think the government should promote a campaign to get people (during ages 40–50) to consent to such research." *Lukas Kalinke, consultation respondent*

"When he still had capacity, my husband consented to take part in lots of research, but he actually became traumatised by over-testing." *Barbara Pointon, consultation respondent*

8.28 A second position is the principle that people should only be involved in research if they had, in the past, expressed a positive desire to participate, for example through some form of advance decision or statement of values. Such a decision might be specific (for example limited to observational research, or research on treatment which has reached a particular stage of testing), or it might be quite general, expressing a general altruistic willingness to participate in any relevant research that has been approved by the appropriate authorities. This approach found significant support in our consultation responses, a number of which highlighted the possible benefits of open discussion of attitudes to research around the time of diagnosis, with the person's opinions about research being clearly documented at the time.[444] It was noted, though, that such advance consent should not automatically give a 'green light' to research, as it may be hard to predict the effect of the research on the person and may cause unforeseen distress. Clearly, our discussion in Chapter 5 as to the way past and present wishes should be balanced (see paragraphs 5.24–5.32) is highly relevant also in relation to research.

Various forms of proxy consent

"[Research should be allowed] only after careful consideration and if it was in accordance with past wishes in an advance directive or they had appointed a person such as a spouse, son or daughter to make that decision for them." *Falkirk Branch – Alzheimer Scotland, consultation respondent*

"Patients are more likely to agree to non-therapeutic research than their carers who I think are naturally defensive. Conversely, carers are more likely to be enthusiastic about intervention and treatment studies, whereas patients are often more reluctant because of fear of adverse effects, or simply 'being changed' by the treatment." *Anonymous consultation respondent*

---

[443] Nuffield Council on Bioethics (2009) *Dementia: Ethical issues – summary of public consultation* (London: Nuffield Council on Bioethics), Q30.
[444] *Ibid.*

8.29 A third option is that of proxy consent. A proxy might be named by the individual in advance of any loss of capacity, or by others at the time the decision is needed. Alternatively, it has also been suggested that a proxy could be named by the individual at the time the consent is required, in circumstances where the individual no longer has capacity to give valid consent to the research proposal but does have the capacity to nominate a trusted person to make the decision.[445] Where a proxy approach is adopted, much will depend on the constraints (if any) placed on the proxy decision maker. Those respondents who commented on the role of a proxy decision maker generally saw it as a positive safeguard, based both on the proxy's prior knowledge of the person's likely approach to research and on the trusted nature of the relationship. It was also highlighted that at present a welfare attorney in England and Wales does not have specific power to give or withhold consent to research (see paragraph 8.34 for a summary of the legal position).[446]

8.30 This positive attitude to proxy consent was not universal, with at least one respondent to our consultation expressing concerns about a proxy's ability to second-guess the wishes of the person with dementia.[447] As we discuss in Chapter 5, however, while there is some evidence to suggest that proxies do not always correctly predict what a person would choose in a particular situation,[448] for many this may not be the key factor. Rather, in nominating a welfare attorney, the person is trusting the nominated individual to make a decision on their behalf in the context of that trusting relationship.

Current legal safeguards

8.31 The law in the UK broadly adopts a proxy-based approach, but imposes varying constraints on the proxy decision maker depending both on the type of research and on where in the UK the research is taking place. A distinction is made between a 'clinical trial' (which aims to test the safety and the effectiveness of a new medicinal product) and other types of research. Clinical trials are regulated by the Clinical Trials Regulations[449] (which apply to the whole of the UK), while other forms of research are regulated in England and Wales by the Mental Capacity Act and in Scotland by the Adults with Incapacity (Scotland) Act. There is as yet no equivalent Act in Northern Ireland (although one is promised for 2011),[450] and hence research in Northern Ireland which does not count as a clinical trial is currently subject to the common law. All medical research involving human participants in the UK must also be approved by an independent research ethics committee.

8.32 All three sets of statutory requirements (the Clinical Trials Regulations, the Mental Capacity Act and the Adults with Incapacity (Scotland) Act) specify criteria that aim to protect people who lack capacity from undue risks in research. All three also require some form of consent from, or consultation with, a proxy. However, there are some differences both in language and in approach between the three pieces of legislation.

[445] See, for example, Kim SYH and Appelbaum PS (2006) The capacity to appoint a proxy and the possibility of concurrent proxy directives *Behavioural Sciences and the Law* **24**: 469–78.

[446] Nuffield Council on Bioethics (2009) *Dementia: Ethical issues – summary of public consultation* (London: Nuffield Council on Bioethics), Q30.

[447] John Shore, responding to the Working Party's consultation.

[448] Ditto PH, Danks JH, Smucker WD *et al.* (2001) Advance directives as acts of communication *Archives of Internal Medicine* **161**: 421–30.

[449] Full title: Medicines for Human Use (Clinical Trials) Regulations 2004, SI 1031, as amended.

[450] Northern Ireland Department of Health, Social Services and Public Safety (2009) *Legislative Framework for Mental Capacity and Mental Health Legislation in Northern Ireland: A policy consultation document* (Belfast: Northern Ireland Department of Health, Social Services and Public Safety), paragraphs 1.4 and 5.3.

8.33 On protecting the individual from harm:

- The Clinical Trials Regulations specify that there must be grounds to expect that administering the product to a person who lacks capacity will produce a benefit to the person that "outweighs" the risks, or will result in no risk at all.

- The Mental Capacity Act requires that research involving incapacitated adults must *either* have the potential to benefit the person without exposing them to "disproportionate" risks, *or*, if no direct personal benefit is expected, the risks must be "negligible" and anything done to the person must not be "unduly invasive or restrictive" or interfere significantly with their freedom of action or privacy.

- The Adults with Incapacity (Scotland) Act requires that the research should involve "only a minimal foreseeable risk" and only "minimal discomfort." The Adults with Incapacity (Scotland) Act adds a further proviso that if the research is not likely to benefit the individual directly, it can go ahead only if it is likely substantially to further scientific understanding, and hence improve care for others (in the future) with the same incapacity. Unlike the Mental Capacity Act, the Adults with Incapacity (Scotland) Act thus sets the same threshold for risk regardless of whether or not the research is likely to benefit the individual.

8.34 On seeking consent:

- In research governed by the Clinical Trials Regulations, consent must be given, either by individuals themselves before loss of capacity, or by a "legal representative." In England, Wales and Northern Ireland, the legal representative may be a suitable relative or friend of the individual, or, if no such person is available, the individual's own doctor as long as he or she is not involved in the research. In Scotland, the first choice of representative is the welfare attorney or guardian, if one has been appointed; if not, it would be the nearest relative, or the individual's own doctor as long as he or she is not involved in the research.

- Under the Mental Capacity Act, however, formal consent is not sought from a proxy: instead, a carer (or other unpaid person interested in the welfare of the person with dementia) must be consulted for advice as to whether the person should take part in the project. If the carer's advice is that the person would not have wished to be involved in the research project, then the person should not be involved. If there is no appropriate unpaid carer to consult, then a person unconnected with the research must be nominated to take on this role. The person's welfare attorney (where one has been appointed) does not have any special role in research decisions, although it is likely that such an attorney would be an obvious choice as the person to be consulted as the 'carer.'

- Under the Adults with Incapacity (Scotland) Act, consent must be obtained from the individual's guardian or welfare attorney or (if no such person has been appointed) from the nearest relative.

8.35 The ethical difficulties inherent in carrying out research among participants with impaired capacity to consent to their involvement has also been addressed by member states of the Council of Europe, through an additional protocol to the 'Oviedo Convention' on human rights and biomedicine (see Box 8.1).[451]

---

[451] Council of Europe (2005) *Additional Protocol to the Convention on Human Rights and Biomedicine, Concerning Biomedical Research* **25 Jan** (Strasbourg: Council of Europe) available at: http://conventions.coe.int/Treaty/en/Treaties/Html/195.htm.

> **Box 8.1: Additional Protocol to the Convention on Human Rights and Biomedicine, concerning Biomedical Research – Article 15**
>
> 1. Research on a person without the capacity to consent to research may be undertaken only if all the following specific conditions are met:
>   i. the results of the research have the potential to produce real and direct benefit to his or her health;
>   ii. research of comparable effectiveness cannot be carried out on individuals capable of giving consent;
>   iii. the person undergoing research has been informed of his or her rights and the safeguards prescribed by law for his or her protection, unless this person is not in a state to receive the information;
>   iv. the necessary authorisation has been given specifically and in writing by the legal representative or an authority, person or body provided for by law, and after having received the information required by Article 16, taking into account the person's previously expressed wishes or objections. An adult not able to consent shall as far as possible take part in the authorisation procedure. The opinion of a minor shall be taken into consideration as an increasingly determining factor in proportion to age and degree of maturity;
>   v. the person does not object.
> 2. Exceptionally and under the protective conditions prescribed by law, where the research has not the potential to produce results of direct benefit to the health of the person concerned, such research may be authorised subject to the conditions laid down in paragraph 1, sub-paragraphs ii, iii, iv, and v above, and to the following additional conditions:
>   i. the research has the aim of contributing, through significant improvement in the scientific understanding of the individual's condition, disease or disorder, to the ultimate attainment of results capable of conferring benefit to the person concerned or to other persons in the same age category or afflicted with the same disease or disorder or having the same condition;
>   ii. the research entails only minimal risk and minimal burden for the individual concerned; and any consideration of additional potential benefits of the research shall not be used to justify an increased level of risk or burden.
> 3. Objection to participation, refusal to give authorisation or the withdrawal of authorisation to participate in research shall not lead to any form of discrimination against the person concerned, in particular regarding the right to medical care.

Are these safeguards appropriate?

8.36 We sought views through our various consultative activities as to whether the current safeguards, described above, are sufficient to protect the individual, or whether, on the contrary, they are seen as unnecessarily hindering research which could be of positive benefit to people with dementia both now and in the future. While the self-selected nature of our consultation respondents prevents the outcomes of the consultation from being presented as fully representative research, we did receive responses from a large number of funding bodies and of individual academics with personal experience of carrying out research. Despite the differences in language between the systems in England and Wales, in Scotland and in Northern Ireland, it was not suggested to us that any particular system was superior to any other, although the practical point was noted that the different systems do not facilitate UK-wide research.[452] Given the current political pressure for more collaboration at European level, this concern may have wider resonance.[453]

8.37 Perhaps unsurprisingly, a number of academic respondents highlighted what they saw as the 'cumbersome' elements of research review, suggesting that increasing requirements for 'form filling and red tape' may be slowing progress and discouraging researchers from developing new models of research.[454] Procedures exist in order to protect and promote the welfare of those with impaired capacity and not for the convenience of researchers; but at the same time it must be recognised that procedures created with the best of intentions may have undesirable consequences and may even defeat their own purposes. Three aspects of the current regulatory position seemed to us to be worthy of particular consideration.

8.38 First, a number of people drew to our attention the fact that research which carries almost no risk of harm to the individual, such as observational research carried out in care homes with the aim of

---

[452] Medical Research Council, and Economic and Social Research Council, responding to the Working Party's consultation.

[453] European Commission press release (2009) *Commission steps up action on Alzheimer's disease and other neurodegenerative conditions* 22 July, available at: http://europa.eu/rapid/pressReleasesAction.do?reference=IP/09/1171&format=HTML&aged=0&language=EN&guiLanguage=en.

[454] Nuffield Council on Bioethics (2009) *Dementia: Ethical issues – summary of public consultation* (London: Nuffield Council on Bioethics), Q31.

improving quality of care, is subject to exactly the same procedures as much more interventionist research.[455] Thus researchers are required to justify to research ethics committees why they wish to amend standard procedures, such as the 'cooling off' period before the research can start, which may be inappropriate in more advanced dementia, where potential participants may have little recall of discussions several days earlier.

8.39 Secondly, there is the question of the *detail* required when providing information to potential participants. It is clearly important in any kind of research that people being invited to take part and those concerned with their welfare have sufficient information on which to make their decision. However, the provision of complex and detailed information, relating not only to the clinical aspects of the research but also to the requirements of data protection legislation, may simply become an intimidating barrier to research and disempower people with dementia altogether from the process. Working Party members' own experience suggests that people with dementia who do not have a keen and committed carer may simply be excluded from the opportunity to participate in research. Moreover, the nature of the material produced may itself determine whether the person with dementia is considered to have capacity to make their own decision (if necessary with support). The detailed information currently required by research ethics committees can exclude people with dementia who are in fact quite capable of understanding the broad concept of a study and of giving their own consent.

8.40 Thirdly, it is of concern that, at present, there is a lack of clarity about the procedures to be followed if a person gradually loses capacity to consent to their ongoing involvement in a research project during that project. In a clinical trial governed by the Clinical Trial Regulations, a person's consent to participate in the trial remains valid after loss of capacity, as long as the trial is not significantly altered.[456] However, the position is more complicated in research which is not a clinical trial.

8.41 In its guidance to researchers, the Medical Research Council notes that neither the Mental Capacity Act nor the Adults with Incapacity (Scotland) Act explicitly set out what should happen if a person loses capacity to consent to their continuing involvement in a research project, with the exception of special provisions governing research that had already begun at the point when the Mental Capacity Act first came into force.[457] The Medical Research Council therefore suggests that, when designing studies, researchers should discuss the possibility of loss of capacity with research participants and include an option to consent to remain within the study in the event of incapacity. This consent would not, however, be absolute, as the person's continued participation would be subject to the Mental Capacity Act or Adults with Incapacity (Scotland) Act safeguards described above (see paragraph 8.34).

8.42 This lack of legal clarity (and hence the increased risk that people who have given consent to take part in research may have to drop out of the project) is of particular concern in dementia, given the degenerative nature of the condition and the risk that the results of studies may be seriously distorted by the withdrawal of participants as they lose the capacity to consent to ongoing participation. If a person who lacks capacity to decide for themselves on their involvement in research shows distress at possible involvement, there is a strong justification, in terms of respecting both their autonomy and well-being, in withdrawing that person from the research. If, on the other hand, the person does *not* appear to experience any distress at the involvement, and had in the past actively chosen to participate, then respect for their autonomy interests would suggest that they should be enabled to continue.

---

[455] See, for example, consultation responses by Alzheimer's Research Trust and the Ethox Centre. The same point arose in the Working Party's fact-finding meeting with Professor Dawn Brooker of the Bradford Dementia Group, 30 Sept 2008.

[456] Schedule 1, Parts 1 and 3, The Medicines for Human Use (Clinical Trials) Regulations, SI 2004/1031, as amended; Medical Research Council (2007) *MRC Ethics Guide: Medical research involving adults who cannot consent* (London: MRC), p15.

[457] Medical Research Council (2007) *MRC Ethics Guide: Medical research involving adults who cannot consent* (London: MRC), pp15–7.

Our approach

8.43 We have argued above that a key way in which solidarity for those with dementia can be expressed is in the promotion of research which seeks to minimise the negative effects of dementia (see paragraph 8.15). Much dementia research requires participants who themselves have dementia, and dementia can affect the ability of people to give valid consent to take part in research. For this reason, dementia research can be held back through the lack of an adequate number of people who are able to consent to take part in research.

8.44 There are clearly good ethical reasons, based on concern for people's autonomy and well-being, for ensuring that strong safeguards are in place to protect people who lack capacity from being harmed by research. Even where a person has expressed an interest in participating in research in the past, concern about their current well-being may in some circumstances make it quite inappropriate for them to be included in a particular research project. However, at the same time there is a risk that, if the procedural bar is set too high, people with dementia will be excluded altogether from research. This, in turn, would be discriminatory: it would prevent people with dementia from acting altruistically when they have autonomously expressed a wish to do so, and would reduce the chance of better treatment and care both now and in the future. **We believe that the current legal safeguards set out in paragraphs 8.31–8.35 above are an appropriate way of protecting people with dementia from harm. However, we believe that action should be taken to make it easier to allow those who have expressed a wish to take part in research to do so.** In particular, we highlight the following:

■ The importance of good clinical trial networks. We have been impressed by networks such as DeNDRoN (see paragraph 8.19) which bring together both clinicians and people with dementia who are interested in helping with clinical trials of promising interventions. Ways of involving more clinicians and patients in these and related networks should be sought.

■ We also emphasise the importance of researchers carefully considering the possible effects of the trial on the person with dementia *beyond* the end of the trial period. Participation in a trial has the potential significantly to affect a person's future well-being or options: for example, those who participated in research on a possible vaccine for Alzheimer's disease will no longer be able to participate in trials of other new medicines. Other examples cited to us of post-trial problems included a case where the person with dementia benefited from a lower dose of the trial drug, but had to be withdrawn from the trial (with adverse effects on his cognition) because he could not tolerate the higher dose being tested.[458]

■ Advance decisions and advance care planning have been given a clear legal status in England and Wales in the Mental Capacity Act. We believe that this focus on future planning also provides a way in which people, while they have the capacity to do so, can state their views and wishes regarding their participation in research at a time in the future when they may lack capacity. Such views and wishes could, with appropriate safeguards, provide a basis for participation in research at a time when the person lacks capacity to consent.

■ While welfare attorneys in Scotland have the power to consent to research on behalf of the person for whom they hold the power of attorney, those in England and Wales do not; instead a carer must be 'consulted' (see paragraph 8.34). It is not clear to us why the power of welfare attorney is restricted in this way in England and Wales.

---

[458] Example cited by one of our peer reviewers.

Recommendation 18: We recommend that the UK Departments of Health should commission research on the feasibility of developing some form of (non-binding) advance statement on research participation which could influence decisions on research participation after loss of capacity.

Recommendation 19: We recommend that serious consideration be given to enable the role of the welfare attorney in England and Wales to be explicitly extended to include decisions over research, both within the Mental Capacity Act and the Clinical Trials Regulations. In the meantime we recommend that the Mental Capacity Act Code of Practice should provide guidance on the role of the welfare attorney in decisions about participation in research governed by the Mental Capacity Act.

Recommendation 20: We further recommend that the mental capacity Codes of Practice should include clear guidance on the procedures to be followed when capacity is lost during involvement in a research project covered by the Act, to minimise the risk of research results being compromised as a result of people dropping out of research despite their initial wish to participate.

8.45 The general *principles* of research governance and consent are, we believe, broadly correct. The *practice*, however, can place unnecessary barriers in the way of research in dementia. In particular:

- The bureaucratic procedures around research ethics approval can be cumbersome for researchers. We encourage current attempts by the Department of Health to simplify the procedures particularly in the context of low-risk research.[459]
- The ability of people with dementia to give, or withhold, valid consent to research should not be underestimated. The information provided both in written and verbal form, however, may need to be provided in a different form for people with some cognitive impairment compared with people without such impairment. Both researchers and ethics committees should adapt the informing process in a way to enable, rather than to exclude, people with dementia in making a valid decision as to whether or not to participate in research.

---

[459] Department of Health (2006) *Best Research for Best Health: A new national health research strategy* (London: Department of Health), paragraph 1.6.

Concluding remarks to the Report

Dementia touches almost all of us. It is so common amongst those who live into old age that there are few families that have no experience of the condition. Most people in the UK with dementia are living in their own home. Many of the residents of care and nursing homes have dementia. As the condition develops, people with dementia are likely to become heavily dependent on the care of others. Those who provide such care – family, friends, professionals and care workers – may face many difficulties because caring can be both physically and emotionally demanding. In addition, carers frequently struggle with ethical problems – with the question of what is the right thing to do. These problems are not limited to end of life care. They can arise day-to-day, in the small details of care, in the apparently mundane. But they are not trivial. On the contrary, they can confront those providing care with stressful dilemmas; and the way in which these ethical difficulties are approached can impact significantly on the lives of people with dementia.

There are laws, guidelines and policies that may articulate a structure that goes some way towards answering the problems which carers face. But usually the problems are so embedded in the human details of the situation, in the exact circumstances and in the nature and history of relationships, that laws and guidelines can provide no more than a sketch of an answer. Indeed, guidelines can sometimes become a hindrance to good care if they lead to a 'tick-box' culture that is too crude an approach to the complexity of the ethical problems, and that dehumanises the relationships and the care. Policies, and the methods by which they are enforced, may focus so much on one issue that they prevent carers from giving due weight to other considerations. 'Risk management' is one example where the concern to prevent putting a person with dementia at any risk may, in some instances, be bought at too great a cost to freedom and quality of life.

The main messages of this Report are that those supporting and caring for people with dementia face ethical problems in carrying out day-to-day care, that these problems are important and stressful, that those providing care receive little support in tackling them, and that providing such support will improve dementia care. We give many examples of the kinds of ethical problems we have in mind. These include: balancing risks and freedom; avoiding telling the truth to prevent distress; the timing and communication of diagnosis; and how to manage conflict between caring for the person with dementia and other commitments.

Our main recommendation is that ethics support to those providing care should be a component of any comprehensive dementia strategy. In Chapter 2 we outline a set of values and methods of ethical analysis that will, we hope, be helpful to those providing care, to those supporting or managing them, and to those involved in education and training. We apply these values and methods to the issues that we discuss throughout the rest of the Report. In other Chapters we give examples of the provision of support that have come to our notice during the consultation process that has informed this report. We have described some of these in the hope that they may lead to further and more widespread improvements in support, recognising the enormous stresses that many carers face on a daily basis.

There are no easy answers to many of the ethical problems that arise for those providing care, and indeed for society more generally, as a result of dementia. Progress in tackling these problems will, we believe, result from increasing awareness coupled with thoughtful support for those who face such problems. Careful analysis of the issues using ethical values and case comparisons will be an important component in providing such support. But analysis alone is not sufficient. It is also crucial that we use our imaginations to understand the experiences and situations both of those with dementia and of their carers. Ian McEwan wrote that "imagining what it is like to be someone other than yourself is at the core of our humanity. It is the essence of compassion, and it is the beginning of morality."[460] While we can never fully imagine or appreciate the impact of another's experience, endeavouring to do so helps in the development of compassion and morality, and informs the analysis of the ethical issues that arise in the setting of dementia.

---

[460] McEwan I (2001) Only love and then oblivion. Love was all they had to set against their murderers *Guardian* 15 Sept, available at: www.guardian.co.uk/world/2001/sep/15/september11.politicsphilosophyandsociety2.

Appendices

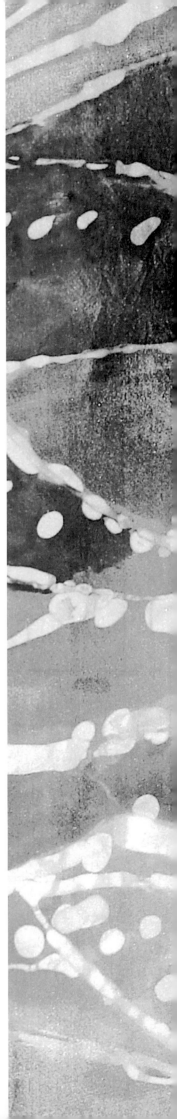

Appendix 1: Method of working

Background

The Nuffield Council on Bioethics examines ethical issues raised by new developments in biological and medical research. In May 2006, the Council held a workshop that addressed ethical issues raised by advances in neuroscience. Following this meeting, the Council concluded that any future work in the area would need to focus on a specific aspect of the subject. Subsequently, the Council decided that it should establish a Working Party to examine the ethical issues raised by degenerative neurological diseases which result in dementia, and so a further workshop was organised, and a Working Party was formed to address ethical issues relating to dementia. The Working Party held its first meeting in November 2007, and had eight further meetings over a period of 17 months.

Consultation document

From May to July 2008, the Working Party held a public consultation which received a higher level of response than any of the Council's previous consultations. Two hundred responses were received from individuals and organisations and, in addition, many people with dementia contributed to group responses by national organisations such as the Alzheimer's Society (England, Wales and Northern Ireland) and Alzheimer Scotland, and to local dementia support groups such as Alzheimer Cafés and Alzheimer associations throughout the UK. Major professional bodies and research charities with an interest in dementia also gave us the benefit of their expertise. While consultation responses cannot necessarily be representative of all those concerned personally or professionally with dementia, they still constitute a considerable body of knowledge and expertise, and this has contributed significantly to the considerations of the Working Party. Moreover, the responses we received to questions about the experiences of living with dementia correspond very closely with the results of research carried out by academics and voluntary organisations in this field. In such cases, we have felt fully justified in placing great weight on the information gained through the consultation exercise.

A list of respondents is available at Appendix 2, and a summary of the consultation is accessible on the Council's website.[461]

Fact-finding

As part of its work, the Working Party held a series of 'fact-finding meetings' with people with direct experience of living with dementia and with those working in the field of dementia.

Meeting with people working at the 'front line' of dementia

On 10 July 2008, the Working Party invited people working at the 'front-line' of dementia – including carers, physicians, people working in social care, legal experts, and ethicists – to comment on various aspects of the issues raised in the consultation. Those who presented at this meeting were:

Chris Belcher
Partner in the Private Client Team at Farrer & Co LLP Solicitors specialising in elder client and Court of Protection matters; Director of Solicitors for the Elderly.

Dr Ron Berghmans
Faculty of Health, Medicine and Life Sciences, Maastricht University.

---

[461] See: http://nuffieldbioethics.org/go/ourwork/dementia/introduction.html.

Claire Biernacki

Nurse and dementia day services manager; author of 'Dementia: Metamorphosis in care'.

Professor Roger Brownsword

Director of the Centre for Technology, Ethics & Law in Society (TELOS), School of Law, King's College London; Council member.

Professor Wim Dekkers

Associate Professor, Philosophy of Medicine, Radboud University Nijmegen Medical Centre.

Dr Gillie Evans

GP for 50 patients with moderate and severe dementia residing in a care home; founder member of a local multidisciplinary Palliative Care in Dementia Group.

Naomi Harris

Social worker, Older Adults' Team, London Borough of Barnet.

Tembi Hlalakuhle

Manager of specialist dementia care home.

Dr Neil Manson

Senior lecturer in philosophy, Lancaster University.

Dr Rupert McShane

Old age psychiatrist, with research interests in GPS tracking for people with dementia; clinical trials; neuroleptics in dementia; pharmacoeconomics; and quality of life in dementia.

Alison Murray

Regulation Manager, 'SOFI' Lead,[462] Commission for Social Care Inspection, South West Regional Office.

Barbara Pointon

Carer for 16 years; member of External Reference Group for the National Dementia Strategy; campaigner for a better deal for people with dementia and their carers.

Frances Swaine

Partner, with a special interest in health care issues, at Leigh Day and Co., solicitors.

Dr Daphne Wallace

Retired psychiatrist working for many years with older people, now with a diagnosis of vascular dementia.

Meetings with members of the Bradford Dementia Group

Professor Tony Hope, Dr Julian Hughes, Dr Jim Eccles, and Katharine Wright met with Professor Murna Downs, Dr Clive Baldwin, and Andrea Capstick from the Bradford Dementia Group on 29 June 2008.

A separate meeting was held on 30 September 2008 with Professor Dawn Brooker from the Bradford Dementia Group, Professor Tony Hope, and members of the Secretariat.

---

[462] SOFI is an abbreviation of 'Short observation framework for inspection', a new inspection technique which involves observing how people with dementia behave and how well staff engage with them, in order to obtain information from people who cannot otherwise communicate with inspection staff.

Visit to Vale House, Oxford

On 30 September, Professor Tony Hope, and members of the Secretariat visited Vale House, a purpose-built specialist care home, caring for 20 people with dementia. They met with Tricia O'Leary (Head of Vale House), Moira Deane (Deputy Head of Home), Evelyn Wilks (Trustee), and Nicky Gale (Family Support Worker).

Visit to an Alzheimer Café in Farnborough

Professor Tony Hope and Dr Gemma Jones visited the Farnborough Alzheimer Café in order to speak to people with dementia and their carers in an informal, social context.

Deliberative event

In addition to its general consultative activities, the Working Party also sought the opinions of people who do not have direct experience of dementia. To achieve this, a one-day 'deliberative event' was held in Birmingham, involving over 50 members of the public, selected to be broadly representative of the age groups and social and ethnic mix found in the UK as a whole. Participants received background information about dementia, and then discussed a number of ethical problems in five smaller groups.

While, again, the information we gained from this event cannot be held to be representative of the whole population, the way the groups tackled the problems, and the remarkable consistency of some of the conclusions (both between the different groups on the day and when considered alongside the responses to the written consultation) were very helpful as we considered both how to formulate our ethical approach, and how some of the specific problems might best be tackled.

Peer review

An earlier version of the Report was peer reviewed by nine individuals with expertise in the areas covered. These were: Professor George Agich; Professor Carol Brayne; Professor Peter Coleman; Professor John Keady; Ms Penny Letts; Dr Stephen Louw; Professor John O'Brien; Mrs Barbara Pointon; and Dr Daphne Wallace.

The Working Party is extremely grateful to all those who took the time to contribute to its work, and for their help in clarifying some of the most challenging issues raised by this Report.

Appendix 2: Wider consultation for the Report

The consultation document

The Working Party published its consultation document[463] on 14 May 2008 and welcomed responses until 31 July 2008.

The document contained six broad themes:

- What is dementia and how is it experienced?;
- Person-centred care and personal identity;
- Making decisions;
- Aspects of care and support;
- The needs of carers; and
- Research.

There were a number of questions within each theme, and background information was provided to clarify some of the issues being addressed. The document was disseminated to individuals and organisations with an interest in any or all of the issues raised by the consultation. Hard copies of the document were posted to more than 1,000 recipients, and it was also made available online. The consultation received coverage in both local and national media.[464]

As well as the main consultation document, respondents were offered a shorter version, and also large-print versions of both the shorter and the full-length documents.

Responses

In all 200 responses were received by the Secretariat and circulated to the Working Party. Of these 200 responses, approximately 70 per cent were from individuals, 23 per cent from organisations, and seven per cent from organisations that arranged events where the consultation document could be discussed by participants.

The responses totalled more than 1,500 pages and provided the Working Party with an invaluable insight into the perspectives of many people closely concerned with dementia. While the respondents did not constitute a representative view of all those with direct experience of dementia, their perspectives and insights were an essential resource for the Working Party in the development of its approach to the final Report. Key themes from the responses have been summarised in a document which is available on the Council's website.[465]

Deliberative event

The Council expanded its usual consultation process to include a one-day workshop with members of the public who had no special knowledge of dementia. Opinion Leader, a research-based consultancy, undertook the organisation and analysis of the event, which took place in Birmingham on 5 August 2008, on behalf of the Council. Fifty four people attended on the day, recruited to form a representative sample of the UK population.

---

[463] See: http://nuffieldbioethics.org/go/ourwork/dementia/page_922.html.
[464] See, for example, BBC News Online (13 May 2008) *Call for debate on dementia care*, available at: http://news.bbc.co.uk/1/hi/health/7398847.stm.
[465] See: http://nuffieldbioethics.org/go/ourwork/dementia/introduction.

The full report and analysis of the deliberative event, produced by Opinion Leader, is available on the Council's website.[466]

List of respondents to the consultation document

Individuals
Anonymous (24)
Ernie Allan
Gillian Andrew
Professor June Andrews, Director, The Dementia Services Development Centre (DSDC), University of Stirling
Norman Ashworth
Tina Auer
Mrs Jacqueline Baldock
Miss Camilla Ball
Margaret Barbour
Claire Biernacki
Susan Boex
Sara Bonfield
Bruce Bovill
Dr Eugene Breen
Dr Guy Brown
Mrs C. Buckle
Jean Burnard
Ross Campbell and Ian Jamieson
H. A. Carsley
Mrs Debra Catton
Mr Keith Chard
Agnes Charnley
Mrs Patricia Clark
Mrs Anne-Marie Clegg
Mrs Kate Copestake
Wendy Cummin
Bill Drake
Jim Ellis, member of the Alzheimer's Society
Mrs Jaki Evans
Annie Foster
Susan M. C. Gibbons
Canon Professor Robin Gill
Beatrice Godwin, Researcher, CDAS, University of Bath
Dr Nori Graham
Miss A. Griffiths
Dr Frank Gunn-Moore
Rt Hon Baroness Hale of Richmond
Barbara Hall
Louise Halloran
Dr Jeremy Harding
Clair Harris

---

[466] *Ibid.*

Mrs Margaret Hawkins

Jonathan Herring

Peter Hindle

Charlie and Margot Hook

Dr Duncan C. S. Hutchison

Colin Isaacs

Dr Ian M. Jessiman

Mrs Kathryn L. Johnston

Professor David A. Jones

Assoc. Professor Robert Jones

Lukas Kalinke

Dr John Kelly

Algy Keuneman

John N. Laurie

Mrs Patricia Laycock

Jan Lethbridge

Moira Livesey

Professor Roberto Llanos

Joseph Loftus

Mrs K. Loughnane

Professor Seth Love

Victoria Main

John Major of Bournemouth

Clive Massey

Professor R. J. Mayer

Nancy McAdam

Dr Hazel McHaffie

Elizabeth McIntyre

Professor Ian McKeith, Newcastle University

Fiona McMurray

Findlay McQuarrie

Angela Melamed

Sally Mendham

Julie Miller

Richard Miller

Miqdad R.

Chreanne Montgomery-Smith

Mrs S. Muller

Mike Newton

Ms Valerie O'Dea

Susan Oliver

Professor Roger Orpwood, Director, Bath Institute of Medical Engineering

Dr Katherine Packham

Mrs Lesley Perrins

Barbara Pointon

Carianne Pudney

Mrs Liz Purcell

Professor Martin Raff

Ms H. Ratokla

Charlotte Rowley

Daphne Sharp
John Shore
Hazel Simpson
Robert Steward
Martin Swann
Professor C. G. Swift
Miss Gill Taylor
Rebecca Taylor
Dr Stephen Ticehurst
Mrs Linda Tolson
Dr C. A. Trotter
Lillian Y. Turner
Mrs G. Tutton
Dr James Warner
David Warren
Chris White
Professor Peter Whitehouse
Professor Gordon Wilcock
Miss Janet Wilkinson
Professor Julie Williams
Mrs D. P. Woodhall
Professor Bob Woods
Mrs Julie Woolgar
A. G. Wright
Ann Yourston

Organisations
AAC Research Unit, University of Stirling
Academy of Medical Sciences
Admiral Nurses – for dementia
Age Concern Camden
Age Concern Leeds
Alzheimer Scotland
Alzheimer's Research Trust
Alzheimer's Society
Alzheimer's Society, South Buckinghamshire Branch
British Geriatrics Society
Bromley PCT
CARE
Christian Council on Ageing; Faith in Elderly People, Leeds
Christian Medical Fellowship
Dementia Services Development Centre (South East), Canterbury Christ
   Church University (Mrs Penny Hibberd, Admiral Nurse/Senior Lecturer)
Department of Palliative Medicine, Velindre Hospital, Cardiff
Dignity in Dying
Ethics Department of the BMA
The Ethox Centre
European Care Group
Falkirk Branch – Alzheimer Scotland
The Field Lane Foundation

Friends of the Elderly
Guideposts Trust
The Inverness Dementia Group
Joseph Rowntree Foundation
The MedicAlert Foundation (Jo Cartwright)
Medical Research Council and Economic and Social Research Council
Mencap
National Prion Clinic
Nursing and Midwifery Council
Office of the Public Guardian (Scotland)
Older People and Disability Team, Social Care and Learning Dept., Bracknell Forest Council
One Creative Environments Ltd.
Poor Servants of the Mother of God
Dr Jacqueline Atkinson, Public Health and Health Policy, University of Glasgow
Royal College of General Practitioners
Royal College of Nursing
Royal College of Physicians
Scottish Dementia Working Group
Scottish Social Services Council
Spiritual Care for Older People (SCOP), Diocese of Oxford
The UK Age Research Forum
United Kingdom Psychiatric Pharmacy Group and The College of Mental Health Pharmacists
The Wellcome Trust

Organisers of events to discuss the consultation document
Carers from Reminiscence Café Drop-in, Memorial Hospital, Oxleas NHS Trust
East Berkshire Alzheimer's Café
Joe's Club, Worcestershire
Leicester University Special Study Group
Stockport Dementia Care Training (Consultation session)
St. Thomas More RC Sixth Form College (Individual participants: Matthew Kevin Ahern, Gemma Bondi, Hollie Gordon, Rachael Hain, Michael Ronan, Adam Rowe, Alexander Thain, Kathryn Whelan)
Westfield School, Newcastle upon Tyne

Appendix 3: Reports by other organisations

Age Concern (2007) *Age of Equality? Outlawing age discrimination beyond the workplace* (London: Age Concern), available at:

www.ageconcern.org.uk/AgeConcern/Documents/ACE_DLR_report_FINAL_PDF.pdf.

Age Concern (2008) *Out of Sight, Out of Mind: Social exclusion behind closed doors* (London: Age Concern), available at:

www.ageconcern.org.uk/AgeConcern/Documents/Out_of_sight_out_of_mind_Feb08.pdf.

All Party Parliamentary Group on Dementia (2008) *Always a Last Resort: Inquiry into the prescription of anti-psychotic drugs to people with dementia living in care homes* (London: Alzheimer's Society), available at:

http://alzheimers.org.uk/downloads/ALZ_Society_APPG.pdf.

All-Party Parliamentary Group on Dementia (2009) *Prepared to Care: Challenging the dementia skills gap* (London: Alzheimer's Society), available at:

www.alzheimers.org.uk/site/scripts/download_info.php?downloadID=329.

Alzheimer Europe (2005) *Comparative Analysis of Legislation in Europe Relating to the Rights of People with Dementia: Final report* (Luxembourg: Alzheimer Europe), available at:

www.alzheimer-europe.org/upload/SPTUNFUYGGOM/downloads/2C8A813C6BBD.pdf.

Alzheimer Europe (2006) *Who Cares? The state of dementia care in Europe* (Luxembourg: Alzheimer Europe), available at:

www.alzheimer-europe.org/upload/SPTUNFUYGGOM/downloads/C9AE88C5E59C.pdf.

Alzheimer's Association (2008) *Voices of Alzheimer's Disease* (Chicago: Alzheimer's Association), available at:

www.alz.org/national/documents/report_townhall.pdf.

Alzheimer Scotland (2003) *Don't Make the Journey Alone* (Edinburgh: Alzheimer Scotland), available at: www.alzscot.org/downloads/dontmake.pdf.

Alzheimer Scotland (2005) *This is my Home: Quality of care for people living with dementia in care homes* (Edinburgh: Alzheimer Scotland), summary available at:

www.alzscot.org/pages/policy/thisismyhome.htm.

Alzheimer Scotland (2009) *Beyond Barriers: Developing a palliative care approach for people in the later stages of dementia: An Alzheimer Scotland partnership project* (Edinburgh: Alzheimer Scotland), available at:

www.alzscot.org/pages/beyond-barriers-palliative-care-report.htm.

Alzheimer's Society (2007) *Home from Home* (London: Alzheimer's Society), available at: http://alzheimers.org.uk/site/scripts/download_info.php?fileID=270.

Alzheimer's Society (2008) *Dementia: Out of the shadows* (London: Alzheimer's Society), available at: http://alzheimers.org.uk/downloads/Out_of_the_Shadows.pdf.

American Academy of Neurology (2001) *AAN Guideline Summary for Clinicians: Detection, diagnosis and management of dementia* (St. Paul, Minnesota: AAN), available at: www.aan.com/professionals/practice/pdfs/dementia_guideline.pdf.

Audit Commission (2004) *Support for Carers of Older People* (London: Audit Commission), available at: www.audit-commission.gov.uk/SiteCollectionDocuments/AuditCommissionReports/NationalStudies/OlderPeople_5_Report.pdf.

Audit Scotland (2008) *A Review of Free Personal and Nursing Care* (Edinburgh: Audit Scotland), available at:
www.audit-scotland.gov.uk/docs/health/2007/nr_080201_free_personal_care.pdf.

The Cabinet Office (2008) *Volunteering in the Public Services: Health & social care – Baroness Neuberger's review as the Government's Volunteering Champion* (London: The Cabinet Office), available at:
www.cabinetoffice.gov.uk/media/cabinetoffice/third_sector/assets/neuberger.pdf.

Care Commission and Mental Welfare Commission for Scotland (2009) *Remember, I'm Still Me* (Edinburgh: Mental Welfare Commission for Scotland; Dundee: Care Commission), available at:
www.carecommission.com/images/stories/documents/publications/reviewsofqualitycare/remember_im_still_me_-_may_09.pdf.

Carers UK (2005) *Caring and Pensioner Poverty: A report on older carers, employment and benefits* (London: Carers UK), available at:
www.carersuk.org/Policyandpractice/Research/Financialimpactofcaring/1207235156/ResearchCaringandpensionerpovertyNovember2005.pdf.

Care Services Improvement Partnership (2007) *Strengthening the Involvement of People with Dementia: A resource for implementation* (London: Department of Health), available at:
www.mentalhealthequalities.org.uk/silo/files/strengthening-the-involvement-of-people-with-dementia.pdf.

Commission for Social Care Inspection (2007) *Rights, Risks and Restraints: An exploration into the use of restraint in the care of older people* (London: CSCI), available at:
www.cambridgeshire.gov.uk/NR/rdonlyres/46979CAB-51B2-4305-B64B-E520165D56D7/0/Restraint.pdf.

Commission for Social Care Inspection (2008) *See Me, Not Just the Dementia: Understanding people's experiences of living in a care home* (London: Commission for Social Care Involvement), available at:
www.cqc.org.uk/_db/_documents/Dementia%20Report-web.pdf.

The Commission on the Future of Volunteering (2008) *Report of the Commission on the Future of Volunteering and Manifesto for Change* (London: The Commission on the Future of Volunteering), available at:
http://www.volunteering.org.uk/NR/rdonlyres/0B8EC40C-C9C5-454B-B212-C8918EF543F0/0/Manifesto_final.pdf.

Dementia Plus (2001) *Twice a Child: Dementia care for African-Caribbean and Asian older people in Wolverhampton* (Wolverhampton: Dementia Plus), available at:
http://www.fordementia.org.uk/assets/files/info_and_support/docs_and_reports/twice-a-child.pdf.

Dementia Services Development Centre, University of Stirling (2006) *The Need to Know: A survey of course input at pre-registration/undergraduate level on dementia* (Stirling: Dementia Services Development Centre).

Department of Constitutional Affairs (2007) *Mental Capacity Act Code of Practice* (London: The Stationery Office), available at:
www.dca.gov.uk/legal-policy/mental-capacity/mca-cp.pdf.

Department of Health (2008) *End of Life Care Strategy: Promoting high quality care for all adults at the end of life* (London: Department of Health), available at:
www.dh.gov.uk/en/Publicationsandstatistics/Publications/PublicationsPolicyAndGuidance/DH_086277.

Department of Health (2009) *Living Well with Dementia: A national dementia strategy* (London: Department of Health), available at:
www.dh.gov.uk/en/Publicationsandstatistics/Publications/PublicationsPolicyAndGuidance/DH_094058.

Driver Vehicle and Licensing Agency (2009) *For Medical Practitioners: At a glance guide to the current medical standards of fitness to drive* (Swansea: Driver and Vehicle Licensing Agency), available at: www.dvla.gov.uk/medical/ataglance.aspx.

Foresight (2008) *Mental Capital and Well-being: Making the most of ourselves in the 21st century – final project report* (London: Government Office for Science), available at: www.foresight.gov.uk/OurWork/ActiveProjects/Mental%20Capital/ProjectOutputs.asp.

HM Government (2008) *Carers at the Heart of 21st Century Families and Communities: "A caring system on your side. A life of your own"* (London: Department of Health), available at: www.dh.gov.uk/en/Publicationsandstatistics/Publications/PublicationsPolicyAndGuidance/DH_085345.

House of Commons Committee of Public Accounts (2008) *Improving Services and Support for People with Dementia* (London: The Stationery Office), available at: http://www.publications.parliament.uk/pa/cm200708/cmselect/cmpubacc/228/228.pdf.

King's Fund (2006) *Securing Good Care for Older People: Taking a long-term view* (London: King's Fund), available at: www.kingsfund.org.uk/research/publications/securing_good.html.

Knapp M and Prince M (King's College London and London School of Economics) (2007) *Dementia UK* (London: Alzheimer's Society), available at: www.alzheimers.org.uk/downloads/Dementia_UK_Full_Report.pdf.

Medical Research Council (2007) *MRC Ethics Guide: Medical research involving adults who cannot consent* (London: Medical Research Council), available at: www.mrc.ac.uk/Utilities/Documentrecord/index.htm?d=MRC004446.

Mental Welfare Commission for Scotland (2006) *Rights, Risks and Limits to Freedom: Principles and good practice guidance for practitioners using restraint in residential care settings* (Edinburgh: Mental Welfare Commission for Scotland), available at: www.mwcscot.org.uk/web/FILES/Publications/Rights_Risks_web.pdf.

Mental Welfare Commission for Scotland (2007) *Safe to wander?* (Edinburgh: Mental Welfare Commission for Scotland), available at: www.mwcscot.org.uk/web/FILES/Publications/Safe_to_Wander.pdf.

MetLife Foundation (2006) *MetLife Foundation Alzheimer's Survey: What America thinks* (New York: MetLife Foundation), for more information, see: http://www.harrisi.com/news/newsletters/clientnews/2006_MetLife.pdf.

Murphy J, Gray CM and Cox S (2007) *Communication and Dementia: How Talking Mats can help people with dementia to express themselves* (York: Joseph Rowntree Foundation), available at: www.jrf.org.uk/sites/files/jrf/2128-talking-mats-dementia.pdf.

National Audit Office (2007) *Improving Services and Support for People with Dementia* (London: The Stationery Office), available at: www.nao.org.uk/publications/0607/support_for_people_with_dement.aspx.

National Audit Office (2008) *End of Life Care* (Norwich: The Stationery Office), available at: www.nao.org.uk/publications/0708/end_of_life_care.aspx.

National Council for Palliative Care (2008) *Creative Partnerships: Improving quality of life at the end of life for people with dementia: a compendium* (London: National Council for Palliative Care).

National Council for Palliative Care (2009) *Out of the Shadows: End of life care for people with dementia* (London: National Council for Palliative Care).

NHS End of Life Care Programme and National Council for Palliative Care (2008) *Advance Decisions to Refuse Treatment: A guide for health and social care professionals* (Leicester: NHS End of Life Care Programme; London: National Council for Palliative Care), available at: www.adrtnhs.co.uk/pdf/EoLC_DOC.pdf.

NHS Scotland (2008) *Living and Dying Well: A national action plan for palliative end of life care in Scotland* (Edinburgh: The Scottish Government), available at: www.scotland.gov.uk/Resource/Doc/239823/0066155.pdf.

NHS Scotland (2008) *Mental Health in Scotland: Dementia – A national priority summary paper* (Edinburgh: The Scottish Government), available at: www.scotland.gov.uk/Topics/Health/health/mental-health/servicespolicy/dementiadec2008.

NICE/SCIE (2006) *Dementia: Supporting people with dementia and their carers in health and social care,* NICE Clinical Guideline 42 (London: NICE and SCIE), available at: www.nice.org.uk/nicemedia/pdf/CG042NICEGuideline.pdf.

Northern Ireland Department of Health, Social Services and Public Safety (2009) *Legislative Framework for Mental Capacity and Mental Health Legislation in Northern Ireland: A policy consultation document* (Belfast: Northern Ireland Department of Health, Social Services and Public Safety), available at: www.dhsspsni.gov.uk/legislative-framework-for-mental-capacity.pdf.

Office of the Deputy Prime Minister (2004) *Mental Health and Social Exclusion: Social exclusion report* (London: Office of the Deputy Prime Minister), available at: www.socialinclusion.org.uk/publications/SEU.pdf.

Office of the Public Guardian (2008) *Reviewing the Mental Capacity Act 2005: Forms, supervision and fees – consultation paper CP26/08* (London: Ministry of Justice), available at: http://webarchive.nationalarchives.gov.uk/+/www.justice.gov.uk/docs/reviewing-mental-capacity-act.pdf.

Opinion Leader (2008) *Deliberative Workshop on Dementia: A report prepared for the Nuffield Council on Bioethics* (London: Opinion Leader).

Royal College of Physicians (2009) *Advance Care Planning: National guidelines,* concise guidance to good practice number 12 (London: Royal College of Physicians), available at: www.rcplondon.ac.uk/pubs/contents/9c95f6ea-c57e-4db8-bd98-fc12ba31c8fe.pdf.

Scottish Government (2007) *Adults with Incapacity (Scotland) Act 2000 Code of Practice: For persons authorised to carry out medical treatment or research under part 5 of the Act* (Edinburgh: The Scottish Government), available at: www.sehd.scot.nhs.uk/mels/CEL2008_11.pdf.

Scottish Government (2008) *Independent Review of Free Personal and Nursing Care in Scotland: A report by Lord Sutherland* (Edinburgh: The Scottish Government), available at: www.scotland.gov.uk/Resource/Doc/221214/0059486.pdf.

Scottish Intercollegiate Guidelines Network (2006) *Management of Patients with Dementia: A national clinical guideline* (Edinburgh: Scottish Intercollegiate Guidelines Network), available at: www.sign.ac.uk/pdf/sign86.pdf.

UK Clinical Research Collaboration (2006) *UK Health Research Analysis* (London: UK Clinical Research Collaboration), available at: www.ukcrc.org/pdf/UKCRC_Health_Research_Analysis_Report.pdf.

Welsh Assembly Government (2007) *A Strategy for Social Services in Wales Over the Next Decade: Fulfilled lives, supportive communities* (Cardiff: Welsh Assembly Government), available at: http://wales.gov.uk/dhss/publications/socialcare/strategies/fulfilledlives/fulfilledlivese.pdf?lang=en.

Welsh Assembly Government (2009) *National Dementia Action Plan for Wales*, consultation draft (Cardiff: Department for Health and Social Services), available at: http://wales.gov.uk/consultations/healthsocialcare/dementiaactionplan/?lang=en.

World Health Organization (2002) *Toronto Declaration on the Global Prevention of Elder Abuse* (Geneva: World Health Organization), available at: www.who.int/ageing/projects/elder_abuse/alc_toronto_declaration_en.pdf.

Glossary

Acetylcholinesterase: An enzyme that breaks down the neurotransmitter acetylcholine in the brain.

Advance directive/decision: A statement made by people with capacity about how they want to be treated in the future if they become ill and at the same time lack capacity to give or refuse consent.

Alpha-synuclein protein: A small, soluble protein found in the brain. Accumulations of this protein are associated with neuronal damage.

Alzheimer's disease: A degenerative condition of the brain associated with excessive and abnormally folded proteins accumulating in the brain.

Anti-psychotic: A medicine which increases or reduces the effect of naturally occurring chemicals in the brain.

ApoE4: A gene associated with increased susceptibility for late-onset Alzheimer's disease.

Assistive technology: A generic term for technological devices designed to enable independence for disabled or older people.

Beta-amyloid: A protein that accumulates around neurones to form amyloid plaques in the brains of people with Alzheimer's disease.

Binswanger's disease: See Sub-cortical vascular dementia.

Biomarker: Molecules or sets of different molecules that, when detected at a particular level in body fluids or tissues, indicate the presence of a disease.

Cardio-pulmonary resuscitation (CPR): An emergency medical procedure consisting of external cardiac massage and artificial respiration.

Care home: A residential home providing personal care, and in some cases nursing care, in addition to living accommodation.

Carer: Here: a person who spends a significant proportion of their life providing unpaid support to family or friends.

Care worker: A person who is employed to provide care services to people with dementia.

Case law: See common law.

Cerebrospinal fluid: A watery fluid filling the brain ventricles and occupying the space between the membranes that cover the brain and spinal cord.

Cholinesterase inhibitor: A chemical that inhibits the cholinesterase enzyme from breaking down acetylcholine, increasing both the level and duration of action of the neurotransmitter acetylcholine.

Chronic: Referring to a health-related state lasting for a long period of time.

Clinical trial: A medical research process which allows safety and efficacy data to be collected for new drugs or medical devices.

Cognitive behavioural therapy: A type of therapy in which unrealistically negative patterns of thought about the self and the world are challenged in order to alter unwanted behaviour patterns or treat mood-related psychiatric disorders such as depression.

Cognitive impairment: Reduced mental functioning.

Cohort study: A form of longitudinal study used in medicine and social science which uses a designated group of people followed or traced, usually over an extended period of time.

Common law: Law developed through court decisions rather than through legislation.

Computed tomography (CT) scanning: A medical imaging technique to study organs of the body which uses a computer to control the motion of the X-ray source and detectors, processes the data, and produces the image.

Creutzfeldt-Jakob disease (CJD): A communicable progressive disease of the human brain, caused by abnormally folded prion protein, in which the degeneration and loss of neurones result in dementia and loss of mobility.

Dementia care adviser: A person who facilitates access to appropriate care, support and advice for those diagnosed with dementia and their carers.

Dilemma: A situation where a choice has to be made between two incompatible alternatives.

Donepezil: A cholinesterase inhibitor used to treat mild to moderate dementia in Alzheimer's disease.

Empirical: Based on observation or experiment rather than theory.

Epidemiological: Relating to the study of the incidence and distribution of diseases.

Frontal lobe: Each of the paired areas of the brain lying immediately behind the forehead, including areas concerned with behaviour, learning, and voluntary movement.

Frontotemporal dementia: A form of dementia covering a range of conditions including Pick's disease, frontal lobe degeneration and dementia associated with motor neurone disease.

Galantamine: A cholinesterase inhibitor used to treat mild to moderate dementia in Alzheimer's disease.

Glutamate: The most abundant neurotransmitter in the brain involved in transmission of excitatory signals from one neurone to another.

Huntington's disease: A rare hereditary disease of the brain manifested in middle age and characterised by irregular body movements, disturbance of speech, and progressive dementia.

Incidence: The frequency of events (such as the onset of illness) in a population.

Lasting Power of Attorney (LPA): In England and Wales, a nomination by one person ('the donor') of another person ('the attorney') to make decisions on their behalf at a time in the future when the donor may lack the capacity to make those decisions. LPAs may cover both financial and welfare matters. In this Report, we refer only to welfare power of attorney and use the term 'welfare attorney' to cover both welfare LPAs and their equivalent in Scotland.

Lewy body dementia: A form of dementia associated with the build up of proteins particularly alpha-synuclein in characteristic accumulations (Lewy bodies) in brain cells.

Longitudinal research: Research involving information about an individual or group at different times throughout a long period.

Magnetic resonance imaging (MRI): A non-invasive method of imaging different organs of the body, including the brain, that makes use of the different properties of sub-atomic particles in a high intensity magnetic field generated in an MRI scanner.

Memantine: A drug that modifies the action of the neurotransmitter glutamate and is used to treat moderate to severe dementia in Alzheimer's disease.

Memory clinic: A specialist centre for diagnosing dementia.

Mini-Mental State Examination (MMSE): A widely-used eleven-question measure that tests five areas of cognitive ability with a maximum total score of 30.

Multi-infarct vascular dementia: A type of dementia caused by a series of small strokes over time each of which causes brain cells to die in many relatively small areas of the brain.

Multisensory stimulation: A dementia care approach which actively stimulates the senses of hearing, touch, vision and smell.

Neurodegenerative diseases: A collection of diseases resulting in or characterised by degeneration of the nervous system, especially of neurones in the brain.

Neurological: Relating to nerve systems.

Neurone: A cell transmitting nerve impulses.

Neuropsychiatric: Relating to the branch of medicine dealing with mental disorders attributable to diseases of the nervous system.

Neuropsychological: Relating to a scientific discipline that studies the structure and function of the brain in relation to specific behaviours.

Neuroscience: Any or all of the sciences dealing with the structure and function of the nervous system and brain.

Neurotransmitter: A chemical 'messenger' in the brain that relays, amplifies, and modulates signals between a neurone and another cell.

Paradigm: A representative example.

Parkinson's disease: A chronic, progressive neurological disorder characterised by tremor, muscle rigidity, and difficulty in initiating movement.

Person-centred care: The idea that there should be recognition of the 'person' in every individual, however advanced their dementia, and of the central place in dementia care of creating and sustaining meaningful relationships.

Pharmacological: Relating to the branch of medicine that deals with the uses, effects, and modes of action of medicines.

Pick's disease: A progressive dementia associated with the accumulation of tau proteins in the brain. It is characterised by slowly progressing changes in character and social deterioration leading to impairment of intellect, memory and language.

Placebo: Here: a substance with no therapeutic effect used as a control in trials testing new medicines.

Plaque: Here: an abnormal accumulation of protein in the brain.

Post-mortem: After death.

Prevalence: Total number of cases (for example, of a disease) in a population at a given time.

Prion disease: A disease characterised by the accumulation of abnormally folded prion protein, which forms plaques in the brain.

Progressive supranuclear palsy: A degenerative brain disease affecting eye movement, balance, mobility, speech and swallowing.

Proxy: A person authorised to act on behalf of another.

Psychosocial: Relating to the influence of social factors or human interactive behaviour.

Reminiscence therapy: Therapy involving the discussion of past activities, events and experiences with another person or group of people, usually with the aid of prompts such as photographs, household items, other familiar items from the past, music, and archive sound recordings.

Rivastigmine: A cholinesterase inhibitor used for mild to moderate dementia in Alzheimer's disease or in Parkinson's disease.

Single-infarct vascular dementia: A type of dementia resulting from a single stroke that results in death of the brain cells in one, relatively large, area.

SPECT (single-photon emission computed tomography): A technique for imaging the organs of the body, including the brain, using radioactive substances.

Statutory: Required or permitted by legislation.

Sub-cortical vascular dementia: A type of dementia associated with vascular damage that leads to damage to neurones in sub-cortical regions of the brain.

Tau: A protein that may fold abnormally and accumulate in the neurones of the brain, causing 'tangles'.

TDP-43: A protein that may accumulate in neurones of patients with fronto-temporal dementia and motor neurone disease.

Telecare: Uses remote technology to monitor the health of the person and alert an appropriate person where necessary.

Temporal lobe: An area of the cerebral cortex in the brain.

Ubiquitin: A protein in neurones commonly present when abnormally folded proteins accumulate.

Vascular dementia: A stroke or a series of small strokes may cause damage to the network of blood vessels (the vascular system) that transport blood within the brain.

Visuoperceptual: Denoting the ability to interpret visual stimuli.

Visuo-spatial: Denoting the ability to comprehend and conceptualise visual representations and spatial relationships.

Welfare attorney: See Lasting Power of Attorney.

List of abbreviations

AAC	Augmentative and alternative communication
A&E	Accident and emergency
ADL	Activity of daily living
BMA	British Medical Association
CARE	Christian Action Research and Education
CIRCA	Computer Interactive Reminiscence and Conversation Aid
CJD	Creutzfeldt-Jakob disease
CMHT	Community mental health team
CSAN	Caritas Social Action Network
CSF	Cerebrospinal fluid
CSIP	Care Services Improvement Partnership
CT	Computed tomography
DART-AD	Dementia antipsychotic withdrawal trial – Alzheimer's disease
DASNI	Dementia Advocacy and Support Network International
DCP	Dementia Care Partnership
DeNDRoN	Dementias and Neurodegenerative Diseases Research Network
DLB	Dementia with Lewy bodies
DSDC	Dementia Services Development Centre
EFNS	European Federation of Neurological Societies
EvIDem	Evidence Based Interventions in Dementia
FTD	Frontotemporal dementia
GP	General practitioner
HIV	Human immunodeficiency virus
JDI	Joint Dementia Initiative
MMSE	Mini-Mental State Examination
MRC	Medical Research Council
MRI	Magnetic resonance imaging
NEURODEM	Dementias and Neurodegenerative Diseases Research Network in Wales
NHS	National Health Service
NICE	National Institute for Health and Clinical Excellence
PDD	Parkinson's disease dementia
PINC	Palliative Initiatives in Neurological Care

PIR	Presence infra-red
SCIE	Social Care Institute for Excellence
SHIELD	Support at Home – Interventions to Enhance Life with Dementia
SIGN	Scottish Intercollegiate Guidelines Network
SPECT	Single-photon emission computed tomography
WHO	World Health Organization

Index